ADVANCES IN MEDICINE AND BIOLOGY

VOLUME 69

ADVANCES IN MEDICINE AND BIOLOGY

Additional books in this series can be found on Nova's website
under the Series tab.

Additional e-books in this series can be found on Nova's website
under the e-book tab.

ADVANCES IN MEDICINE AND BIOLOGY

VOLUME 69

LEON V. BERHARDT
EDITOR

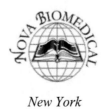

New York

For permission to use material from this book please contact us:
Telephone 631-231-7269; Fax 631-231-8175
Web Site: http://www.novapublishers.com

NOTICE TO THE READER

The Publisher has taken reasonable care in the preparation of this book, but makes no expressed or implied warranty of any kind and assumes no responsibility for any errors or omissions. No liability is assumed for incidental or consequential damages in connection with or arising out of information contained in this book. The Publisher shall not be liable for any special, consequential, or exemplary damages resulting, in whole or in part, from the readers' use of, or reliance upon, this material. Any parts of this book based on government reports are so indicated and copyright is claimed for those parts to the extent applicable to compilations of such works.

Independent verification should be sought for any data, advice or recommendations contained in this book. In addition, no responsibility is assumed by the publisher for any injury and/or damage to persons or property arising from any methods, products, instructions, ideas or otherwise contained in this publication.

This publication is designed to provide accurate and authoritative information with regard to the subject matter covered herein. It is sold with the clear understanding that the Publisher is not engaged in rendering legal or any other professional services. If legal or any other expert assistance is required, the services of a competent person should be sought. FROM A DECLARATION OF PARTICIPANTS JOINTLY ADOPTED BY A COMMITTEE OF THE AMERICAN BAR ASSOCIATION AND A COMMITTEE OF PUBLISHERS.

Additional color graphics may be available in the e-book version of this book.

Library of Congress Cataloging-in-Publication Data

ISBN: 978-1-62808-088-9

ISSN: 2157-5398

Published by Nova Science Publishers, Inc. † New York

Contents

Preface

This continuing series gathers and presents original research results on the leading edge of medicine and biology. Each article has been carefully selected in an attempt to present substantial topical data across a broad spectrum. Topics discussed include prostaglandins and neural function; expression and involvement of cytokines, chemokines and adhesion molecules in rheumatoid vasculitis; understanding soybean rust interaction with soybean using biotechnology; diversity and evolution of fungal phytopathogens associated with snow; the action mechanism, biological effect and clinical significance in improving peripheral arterial blood flow of prostaglandin E1; molecular basis of hemibiotrophy in the lentil anthracnose pathogen colletotrichum truncatum; detection of gaze atypical patterns in Austism Spectrum Disorders; and game-based learning and serious game utilization for people with ADHD.

Chapter I – Prostaglandins are a group of 20-carbon fatty acids produced from arachidonic acid via the cyclooxygenase (COX) pathway in response to extrinsic stimuli. These fatty acids act through specific G-protein-coupled receptors to regulate biological functions such as hormone release, body temperature, cardiovascular activity, inflammation and development. In the nervous system, prostaglandins regulate behaviors such as reduced exploratory activity, decreased locomotion, sedation, convulsions, stupor and catatonia in many species. In goldfish, prostaglandins can synchronize sexual behavior in the opposite sex. Other neural functions such as analgesia, neurotransmitter release, neurogenesis, olfaction, sleep, synaptic plasticity and formation of dendritic spines are also associated with prostaglandins. Arachidonic acid or one of its metabolites can be synthesized selectively within a given cell type initially stimulated by a neurotransmitter and then released into the extracellular space. The compounds can then be metabolized in target cells by specific enzymes. In this mode, prostaglandins can play a diverse role in their attributed neural function. In addition, prostaglandins are involved in many pathological conditions such as autism, cerebral vasospasm and ischemia, migraine, malformations and neurodevelopmental defects. Therefore, understanding the effects and mechanisms of prostaglandins in neural pathogenesis could link to improvements in human health.

Chapter II – Prostaglandin E_1 (PGE_1) is a hormonal compound that shares with other prostaglandin series its origin as a metabolite of polyunsaturated fatty acids, constituent of cell membrane phospholipids, and the diversity of its autocrine and paracrine biological activities. This broad profile of actions ranges from inhibition of the chemiotaxis and the activation of white cells, to profibrinolytic effect and reduction of hematic viscosity. Amongst the pharmacodynamic properties of PGE_1, improvement of the peripheral circulation is probably the most significant of its biological effects. The action is induced by a potent peripheral vasodilation and the inhibition of platelet aggregation and adhesion, mediated by cyclic adenosine-monohophosphate (cAMP). These activities, once it is liberated to the circulation, are mostly loco-regional due to its fast enzyme inactivation, which reaches up to 90% after first lung passage and a half life in plasma of less than two minutes. The chemical stability and hydrophobicity can be improved significantly by complexing PGE_1 to other molecules, like α-ciclodextrin, making it suitable for exogenous administration and therapeutic use. The vasoactive properties of PGE_1 make it a valuable tool for the treatment of peripheral arterial disease and critical limb ischemia in particular, amongst other medical applications. In a clinical situation in which perfusion has been reduced to a point that viability of the limb is dramatically endangered, PGE_1 is the pharmacological treatment of choice in many occasions. This takes place when surgical and endovascular solutions are not an option, failed or as an adjuvant treatment of those therapies, due to its capacity to improve macro and micro circulation. Although traditionally this anti-ischemic action was explained by the combined direct vasodilation and inhibition of platelet function, recent experimental findings suggest that more factors may contribute to its clinical efficacy. This includes anti-inflammatory effects, inhibition of expression of adhesion molecules and generation and release of growth factors, suggesting an improvement in endothelial function and a decrease of vascular cell activation, which could explain the long-term benefits on PGE_1. Its clinical use covers a broad range of ischemic related disorders including peripheral arterial occlusive disease, Reynaud syndrome, scleroderma, Lupus, Buerger´s disease, ergotism, atheroembolic disease, hypertensive ulcers, etc. Because of its rapid inactivation during lung passage, PGE_1 has to be administered either intra-arterial or in large doses intravenous, in order to treat peripheral arterial disease. While intra-arterial applications had been recommended initially, the high rate of secondary effects and complications make intravenous infusions the preferred application route at present. In this chapter the authors will explore the biochemistry, physiological role and therapeutic potential of the PGE_1, along with the latest advances on its use in the treatment of clinical entities involving peripheral ischemia.

Chapter III – Rheumatoid vasculitis (RV) is an uncommon but severe complication of rheumatoid arthritis (RA) that can cause skin disorders, such as rashes, cutaneous ulcerations, gangrene, neuropathy, eye symptoms, and systemic inflammation. Although the molecular mechanisms underlying RV are unclear, it is well known that a chronic imbalance in the expression of chemokines and proinflammatory cytokines facilitates inflammatory responses in RA patients. Dysregulation of cytokines and other inflammatory molecules, such as adhesion molecules, has also been suggested to occur in patients with RV. Recently, the authors reported elevated levels of the chemokine CX3CL1 and macrophage migration inhibitory factor in the serum of patients with RV. In this chapter, the authors discuss the involvement of cytokines and inflammatory molecules in the pathogenesis of RV and evaluate their significance as useful laboratory parameters of active vasculitis disease.

Chapter IV – United States, Brazil and Argentina are the three biggest producers of soybean in the world withat a combined 180 million metric tons each year. Soybean growing in these countries is susceptible to soybean rust caused by *Phakopsora pachyrhizi* Sydow. With new and emerging biotechnological techniques the authors may develop new strategies for broadening resistance of soybean to soybean rust. Using these new techniques, scientists can identify and study genes expressed during a plant-pathogen interaction from the perspective of both plant and pathogen to better understand the infection process. The recent development of techniques, such as microarray analysis, high-throughput DNA sequencing and laser capture microdissection, has dramatically improved our ability to identify new genes and to examine gene expression in small samples. Microarrays can be used to study changes in expression of thousands of genes per experiment in infected leaves. The complete soybean genome sequence now available provides a template for analyzing gene expression results from deep sequencing of transcripts during the infection process. Deep sequencing provides unprecedented amounts of data for analysis of the genome and gene expression. Laser capture microdissection allows the isolation of specific cells from infected leaf cross-sections that can be analyzed for plant and pathogen gene expression using diverse DNA sequencing approaches. There is still a great lack of knowledge of the function of soybean and fungal genes and their spatial and temporal expression. However, these new techniques will provide new information about pathogen development in its host and the host's response to the pathogen. Some of these plant and fungal genes may be useful to broadening soybean resistance to soybean rust.

Chapter V – Cryophilic fungi spend a certain life stage or whole life cycle (sexual and/or asexual reproduction) in the cryosphere where biosphere is constantly or seasonally covered with snow and/or ice. Several groups of cryophilic fungi and their relatives infect other living organisms including fungi. Cryophilic fungal phytopathogens exist in different depths of snow cover, according to their ecophysiological characteristics. Snow fungi represent a fungal group growing on the snow surface, consisting of chytridiomycetes and ascomycete. They are pathogenic to algae growing on the snow. Chytridiomycetes have flagella in a certain stage of their life cycles to reach and infect their hosts, inciting diseases on algae. Snow molds attack overwintering plants within and under snow and include various fungal taxa (mainly oomycetes, ascomycetes and basidiomycetes). Ascomycetous snow molds are pathogenic on the needles of conifers, causing defoliation and blight in snow. They are adapted to xeric conditions and infect hard host tissues such as conifer needles. Herbaceous plants are attacked by a variety of cryophilic fungal phytopathogens under snow where antagonism from mesophilic microorganisms seldom occurs. These fungi are well adapted to the environment where ambient temperature vary at around subzero temperatures. Cyst-like fungal bodies are observed inside fruit bodies of snowbank slime molds (nivicolous myxomycetes). Phylogenetic analyses suggested that they belonged to cryptomycota. In conclusion, cryophilic pathogens are evolved from diverse fungal taxa to adapt to nival environments, developing cold tolerance and selecting host organisms.

Chapter VI – Hemibiotrophic fungal plant pathogens cause enormous economic damage to important food crops, such as cereals, legumes and oil seeds. These pathogens have two distinct *in planta* growth phases, an initial symptomless biotrophic and a subsequent destructive necrotrophic phase where the switch to necrotrophy is critical for disease development. The authors' recent studies indicate that pathogens likely secrete effector proteins to induce a hypersensitive cell death response triggered precisely before the switch to necrotrophy, and this cell death is critical for morphological and genetic differentiation of intracellularly proliferating secondary fungal hyphae. Toxins and hydrolyzing enzymes likely amplify cell death signals to accommodate the pathogen life-style. Here, the authors provide novel insight into the role of effectors in the hemibiotrophic parasitism of *Colletotrichum truncatum*, the causative agent of lentil anthracnose.

Chapter VII – This chapter provides a review on the evolution of the Eye Tracking technology and the use of this technology in the detection of atypical patterns in people with autistic spectrum disorder (ASD). ASDs constitute one of the most serious mental diseases in the chilhood due to the complexity of its detection, diagnosis and treatment, despite the fact that its prevalence is lower than in other chilhood pathologies. For some decades now, the examination of the eye pattern in this collective has begun, due to the fact that they present an alteration in the use of multiple non-verbal behaviours, such as the eye contact. The studies conducted so far have been guided by two types of tests: videos with social /non-social scenes, or with static images. It has been proven the differences between the control groups and the people affected by ASD, and more precisely in those dynamic stimuli including social scenes, in which, the fixing in the eye contours diminishes, thus increasing in the regions or the body or other objects, being this a predictive element of the social response of these people. This chapter discusses the tendencies and results of the use of the Eye Tracking technology carried out to date within the field of the autistic spectrum disorder.

Chapter VIII – This chapter explains the thematic of Serious Games, and specially their application in the field of health and their exploitation within the collective of Attention Deficit Hyperactivity Disorder (ADHD) which is one of the most prevalent childhood disorders. The key point in the development of children diagnosed with ADHD is to enhance motivation and engagement towards academic activities and therapies. *Serious Games for Health* could be a complementary solution constituting a powerful tool that fosters engagement and motivation in therapies combining video game technologies with therapies. Even though some studies are focused on the evidence of possible adverse effects related to the misuse or abuse of videogames in children diagnosed with ADHD; there are videogames that boost and enhance key features in the development of these diagnosed children and teenagers. This chapter gives an historical contextualization of this trend and reviews the markets available, as well as studies its application within the field of the Attention Deficit Hyperactivity Disorder (ADHD) and reviews the trend analysis in this field. As a final conclusion it could be stated that the use game based therapies in junction with other technologies for therapy customization in real time could be an effective way of therapy in its use in children and teenagers diagnosed with ADHD.

In: Advances in Medicine and Biology. Volume 69
Editor: Leon V. Berhardt

Chapter I

Prostaglandins and Neural Functions: A Review

Yu-Wen Chung-Davidson, Ke Li and Weiming Li*

Department of Fisheries and Wildlife,
Michigan State University, US

Abstract

Prostaglandins are a group of 20-carbon fatty acids produced from arachidonic acid via the cyclooxygenase (COX) pathway in response to extrinsic stimuli. These fatty acids act through specific G-protein-coupled receptors to regulate biological functions such as hormone release, body temperature, cardiovascular activity, inflammation and development. In the nervous system, prostaglandins regulate behaviors such as reduced exploratory activity, decreased locomotion, sedation, convulsions, stupor and catatonia in many species. In goldfish, prostaglandins can synchronize sexual behavior in the opposite sex. Other neural functions such as analgesia, neurotransmitter release, neurogenesis, olfaction, sleep, synaptic plasticity and formation of dendritic spines are also associated with prostaglandins. Arachidonic acid or one of its metabolites can be synthesized selectively within a given cell type initially stimulated by a neurotransmitter and then released into the extracellular space. The compounds can then be metabolized in target cells by specific enzymes. In this mode, prostaglandins can play a diverse role in their attributed neural function. In addition, prostaglandins are involved in many pathological conditions such as autism, cerebral vasospasm and ischemia, migraine, malformations and neurodevelopmental defects. Therefore, understanding the effects and mechanisms of prostaglandins in neural pathogenesis could link to improvements in human health.

* Contact Information: Yu-Wen Chung-Davidson: E-mail: chungyuw@msu.edu, Phone: +1 (517) 432-2777.

Introduction

Prostaglandins are a group of 20-carbon fatty acids produced from arachidonic acid via the cyclooxygenase pathway in response to extrinsic stimuli (Smith 1989, 1992; Smith et al., 1991; Smith et al., 2011). Prostanoid biosynthesis (including classical prostaglandins PGD, PGE and PGF, as well as prostacyclins and thromboxanes) proceeds in three stages: (1) extrinsic stimuli-activated mobilization of esterified arachidonate from precursor lipids in the cell membrane through the action of lipases, (2) conversion of arachidonate to the prostaglandin endoperoxide (PGH_2) mediated by PGH synthases, and (3) cell-specific isomerization or reduction of PGH_2 by specific synthases (isomerases) or reductases to the major biologically active prostanoids PGD_2, PGE_2, $PGF_{2\alpha}$, prostacyclin (PGI_2), or thromboxane A_2 (TXA_2; Figure1, modified from Smith, 1992; Smith et al., 2011).

Prostaglandins are local hormones (i.e. autocoids; Smith 1989, 1992; Smith et al., 1991). Infused PGE and PGF derivatives fail to survive a single pass through the circulatory system. Their synthesis is not restricted to a central endocrine organ, but rather occurs in most organs, although not necessarily in all cell types. The plasma concentrations of these compounds, except in rare situations, are less than $10^{-9}M$, a concentration normally unable to elicit responses.

The low plasma concentrations of prostaglandins are a consequence of active catabolism, which begins with oxidation of the 15-hydroxyl group to yield the 15-oxo-derivatives which have 10- to 100-fold less activity than the parent compounds. There are different 15-hydroxyprostaglandin dehydrogenases specific for different prostaglandins (Smith 1989, 1992; Smith et al., 1991). Prostaglandins are ubiquitously distributed in virtually all mammalian tissues and organs (Ito et al., 1992). Prostaglandin levels in snap-frozen samples are generally very low, in the range of ng/g (Wolfe et al., 1976). However, in different species, the predominant prostaglandins may vary (Wolff, 1988).

In the rodent brain, PGD_2 is the major cyclooxygenase metabolite, followed by lower concentrations of $PGF_{2\alpha}$, PGE_2 and PGI_2 (Abdel-Halim et al., 1977; Hayashi et al., 1987; Hertting and Serigi, 1989; Narumiya et al., 1982; Ogorochi et al., 1984; Sun et al., 1977).

In the human neocortex, only a minute amount of PGD_2 was found due to its rapid metabolism into 9α, 11β-PGF_2 (Wolfe, 1988; Wolfe et al., 1989). $PGF_{2\alpha}$ was first thought as the most abundant prostaglandin in human brain (Abdel-Halim et al., 1980a). Later, the presence of prostaglandins D_2, E_2 and $F_{2\alpha}$ was demonstrated *post-mortem* in various regions of the human brain, pineal body and pituitary. Prostaglandins D_2 and E_2 were abundant in pineal body, pituitary, olfactory bulb and hypothalamus. $PGF_{2\alpha}$ was more evenly distributed throughout the human brain (Ogorochi et al., 1984). Therefore, prostaglandins appear to have species-specific and tissue-specific compositions.

Prostaglandins exert powerful central effects on the regulation of behavior, body temperature, cardiovascular activity, and neurotransmitter functions (Chiu and Richardson, 1985). Different members of the prostaglandin family may serve different functions in the brain due to their differential distribution (Abdel-Halim et al., 1980a,b). Both PGD_2 and PGE_2 are implicated in physiological regulation of sleep (Hayaishi, 1988). PGD_2 also exerts neuromodulatory effects on hormone release, body temperature, olfactory function, and analgesia (Ito et al., 1989). Prostaglandins of the E and F series can mediate hyperthermia and fever (Eguchi et al., 1988; Feldberg and Milton, 1978; Lazarus, 2006), as well as neurogenesis (Chung-Davidson et al., 2008b; Uchida et al., 2002). PGE_2 and $PGF_{2\alpha}$ have been implicated in various cerebral functions including the autoregulation of blood flow (Chemtob et al., 1990b). PGE_2 is also involved in inflammation (Hata and Breyer, 2004), development (Li et al., 1993), synaptic plasticity and formation of dendritic spines (Burks et al., 2007; Chen et al., 2002; Zhu et al., 2005).

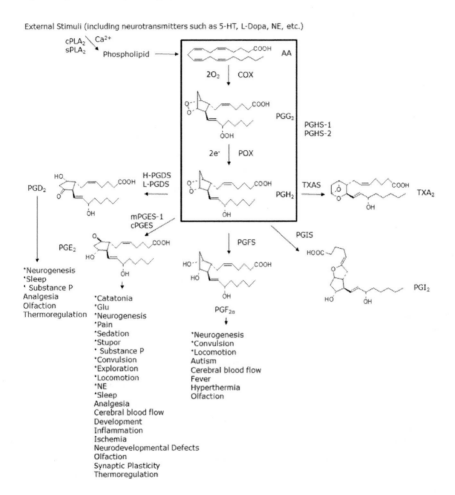

Figure 1. A schematic diagram of the biosynthesis and neural functions of prostaglandins. 5-HT, 5-hydroxytryptamine; AA, arachidonic acid; Glu, glutamate; $cPLA_2$, cytosolic phospholipase A_2; $sPLA_2$, nonpancreatic, secretory phospholipase A_2; PG, prostaglandin; PGHS, prostaglandin endoperoxide H synthase; COX, cyclooxygenase; POX, peroxidase; H-PGDS, hematopoietic PGD synthase; L-PGDS, lipocalin-type PGD synthase; cPGES, cytosolic PGE synthase; mPGES-1, microsomal PGE synthase-1; PGFS, PGF synthase; PGIS, PGI (prostacyclin) synthase; NE, norepinephrine; TXAS, thromboxane A synthase.

This chapter will briefly review the receptors and signal transduction pathways of prostaglandins and the roles of prostaglandins in neural functions such as neurotransmission, neurogenesis, behavior, pain, thermoregulation, and the possible risk of pathogenesis.

Prostaglandins Act through G-Protein Coupled-Receptors

Prostaglandins mediate important physiological functions in the nervous system via activation of G-protein-coupled receptors (Kennedy et al., 1982; Sasaki et al., 1985; Coleman, 1987; Santoian et al., 1989; Abran et al., 1994). Prostanoid receptors are classified into two groups. One group consists of the PGD_2 receptor, the PGE receptor in most tissues (EP_{2-4}), and the PGI_2 receptor, which are linked to cyclic adenosine monophosphate (cAMP) formation (Jumblatt and Paterson, 1991; Sugimoto et al., 1992). The other group comprises the $PGF_{2\alpha}$ receptor, the TXA_2 receptor, and EP_1 (a subtype of PGE receptor) which are linked to phosphoinositol metabolism and Ca^{2+} mobilization (Halushka et al., 1989; Ito et al., 1992; Suba and Roth, 1987).

Prostaglandins can exert diverse neural functions through the activation of different types of receptors and signal transduction pathways. The four G-protein coupled E-prostanoid receptors (EP_{1-4}) are well-characterized prostaglandin receptors. EP_1 is involved in regulation of intracellular calcium levels by the action of phospholipase C (PLC) and inositol 1,4,5-triphosphate (IP_3). EP_2 and EP_4 receptors mediate activation of protein kinase A (PKA) through the action of cAMP and calcium level via different mechanisms, depending on the type of associated G-proteins (Breyer et al., 2001).

Prostaglandins and Neurotransmitters

Several neurotransmitters can modulate prostaglandin release in the brain. 5-hydroxytryptamine (5-HT) enhances the release of prostaglandins (Wolfe et al., 1976; Schaefer et al., 1978). Micromolar concentrations of muscarinic agonists induce the release of PGE_2 and PGF_2 in cerebellar cortical slices (Reichman et al, 1987). However, acetylcholine, in the presence of physostigmine (Hillier et al., 1976), has no effect on prostaglandin release. Catecholamines and L-dopa have an effect on prostaglandin release from central nervous tissues under *in vitro* conditions (Chiu and Richardson, 1985).

Norepinephrine induces PGE_2 release in various rodent brain areas (Hillier et al., 1976, 1979; Schaefer et al., 1978; Schaad, 1989) through the activation of $\alpha 1$-adrenergic receptors (Burch et al., 1986a,b). Higher concentrations of norepinephrine are required to elicit $PGF_{2\alpha}$ release (Wolfe et al., 1976; Schaefer et al., 1978; Hillier et al., 1979; Seregi and Hertting, 1984).

However, the mechanism of $PGF_{2\alpha}$ release may not involve the catecholamine receptor since it is reduced by monoamine-oxidase inhibitors (Schaefer et al., 1978), which are known to inhibit PGI_2 synthesis (Gryglewski et al., 1976). Histamine has no effect on prostaglandin release (Wolfe et al., 1976).

Prostaglandins can also regulate neurotransmitter release. PGE_2 inhibits the release of norepinephrine in the peripheral nervous system and in cortical slices (Hedqvist, 1970; Bergstrom et al., 1973; Reimann et al., 1981; Templeton, 1988) via decrease in Ca^{2+} conductance (Mo et al., 1985). The release of substance P is increased by PGD_2 and PGE_2 in cultured sensory neurons (Vasko et al., 1989). Glutamate release was induced from astrocytes that are important for neuroblast survival and proliferation, and this signal may be accentuated following ischemia or-injury-induced PGE_2 release (Dave et al., 2010). It is conceivable that arachidonic acid or one of its metabolites such as PGH_2, is synthesized selectively within a given cell type initially stimulated by a neurotransmitter and then released into the extracellular space.

The compounds can then be metabolized in target cells by specific enzymes. In this mode, prostaglandins can play a diverse role in their attributed neural functions (Schaad et al., 1991).

Prostaglandins and Behavior

In general, prostaglandins reduce locomotor behavior and induce sleep or stupor in animals. The most common behavioral effects of prostaglandin E series are sedation and the inhibition of locomotor and exploratory activities (Chiu and Richardson, 1985). Interestingly, prostanoids of the A and F series reduce locomotor activity but do not exert sedative effects (Horton and Main, 1965; Gilmore and Shaikh, 1972; Nistico and Marley, 1976). The differences in the pharmacological effects of A, E and F prostanoids may be quantitative (Chiu and Richardson, 1985). The three behavioral effects (reduced exploratory activity, decreased locomotor activity, and sedation) can be viewed as a continuum, such that the least potent agent can be expected to reduce the exploratory activity without affecting the other two parameters, whereas the most potent agent can produce all three behavioral effects. Thus ranked, the prostanoids of the E series are the most potent, while the F series are of intermediate strength, and the A series are the weakest in producing behavioral effects (Chiu and Richardson, 1985).

Prostaglandins of the E series, when injected into the lateral ventricles (i.v.t.) in the cat, produced stupor and catatonia (Horton, 1964). Similar effects were observed after i.v.t. injection of cholinergic agents such as physostigmine and acetylcholine in cats (Feldberg and Sherwood, 1954, 1955) and monkeys (Desijaru, 1973). Since catatonia does not result from either the i.v. or i.p. injection (Horton, 1964; Bloss and Singer, 1978), this effect is localized within the brain (Chiu and Richardon, 1985).

Prostaglandins of the E and F series reduce the debilitating effects of convulsions in animals (Chiu and Richardson, 1985). The level of prostaglandins, in particular of the F type, increases tremendously in the brain during convulsions in animals (Steinhauer et al., 1979) and humans (Egg et al., 1980). Such an increase in prostaglandin release may serve a protective role (Chiu and Richardson, 1985).

PGD_2 plays a role in sleep regulation (Giles and Leff, 1988; Hayaishi, 1989, 2002; Herlong and Scott, 2006; Huang et al., 2007). A single injection of PGD_2 increases the sleeping time in rats or monkeys by 400-600%. In contrast, PGE_2 suppresses slow wave- and REM-sleep while its antagonist reduced the awakening time (Matsumura et al., 1989).

In goldfish, $PGF_{2\alpha}$ plays a dual role as a hormone and a pheromone to synchronize male and female sexual behaviors (Stacey, 1987). At the time of ovulation, female oviducts synthesize and secret $PGF_{2\alpha}$ that induces reproductive behaviors (Stacey and Peter, 1979; Sorensen et al., 1988). $PGF_{2\alpha}$ and its metabolites (mainly 15-keto-$PGF_{2\alpha}$) are also released into water as postovulatory pheromones that induce male spawning behavior and increase male gonadotropin-II and sperm production (Sorensen et al., 1988, 1989; Sorensen and Goetz, 1993). Whether $PGF_{2\alpha}$ is involved in the sexual behavior of other animals has not been investigated.

Prostaglandins and Neurogenesis

Prostaglandins are involved in neurogenesis. The self-renewal and multipotency of neural progenitor cells are regulated by various humoral factors under physiological and pathological conditions such as ischemia (Nakatomi et al., 2002), seizure (Parent et al., 1997), and sleep (Guzmán-Marín et al., 2003). Since PGD_2 is the major cyclooxygenase metabolite in rodents (Abdel-Halim et al., 1977; Hayashi et al., 1987; Hertting and Serigi, 1989; Narumiya et al., 1982; Ogorochi et al., 1984; Sun et al., 1977), and plays a role in sleep regulation (Giles and Leff, 1988; Hayaishi, 1989, 2002; Herlong and Scott, 2006; Huang et al., 2007), it seems to be a good candidate for regulating neurogenesis. Indeed, PGD_2 has been shown to have biphasic effects on neural progenitor cell proliferation (Katura et al., 2010). 15-deoxy-$\Delta^{12,14}$-prostaglandin J_2 (15d-PGJ_2), a nonenzymatic metabolite of PGD_2, regulates progenitor cell proliferation (Katura et al., 2010). 15d-PGJ_2 is endogenously produced from PGD_2 through spontaneous nonenzymatic dehydration followed by isomerization and is an endogenous ligand for peroxisomal proliferator-activated receptor γ (PPARγ) (Forman et al., 1995), which plays a critical role in the regulation of cell differentiation and metabolism (Debril et al., 2001; Walczak and Tontonoz, 2002).

Although the exact mechanisms have yet to be identified, $PGF_{2\alpha}$ induces adult neurogenesis in the diencephalon of goldfish, which is known to be involved in reproduction (Chung-Davidson et al., 2008a,b). $PGF_{2\alpha}$ also induced neurogenesis in several brain regions including the telencephalon and brain stem motor nuclei in goldfish. This is the first evidence that prostaglandin $PGF_{2\alpha}$ can act as a pheromone through the olfactory system to induce neurogenesis in adult brains (Chung-Davidson et al., 2008b).

PGE_2 also regulates the activities of neural progenitor cells (Uchida et al., 2002). Neurogenesis persists in two regions of the adult brain in mammals: the subventricular zone (SVZ) along the lateral ventricles and the subgranular zone of the hippocampal dentate gyrus (Luskin, 1993; Lois and Alvarez-Buylla, 1994). Neurogenesis in the dentate gyrus of adult rodents is elicited by transient global ischemia (Liu et al., 1998; Uchida et al., 2002). COX-2, a rate-limiting enzyme for prostanoid synthesis, is also induced by ischemia (Uchida et al., 2002). Administration of a non-selective COX inhibitor to ischemic animals suppressed cell proliferation in the subgranular zone (SGZ) at the dentate gyrus of the hippocampus (Kumihashi et al., 2001; Uchida et al., 2002). Hippocampal injection of sulprostone, an analogue of PGE_2, increased the number of 5-bromo-2'-deoxyuridine (BrdU)-immunoreactive cells in the SGZ (Uchida et al., 2002). Therefore, PGE_2 may play an important role in cell proliferation in the SGZ (Uchida et al., 2002). PGE_2 exerts its neurogenic effects through four G-protein coupled E-prostanoid receptors (EP$_{1-4}$). EP$_{1-4}$ receptor mRNA levels were elevated during neurogenesis in mouse (Tamiji and Crawford, 2010). PGE_2 may stimulate neurogenesis via EP$_3$ receptors in the dentate gyrus in rodents. However, the involvement of other prostaglandin receptors in neurogenesis remains to be elucidated (Uchida et al., 2002).

Prostaglandins and Pain

Chronic pain involves a mix of both inflammatory and neuropathic processes, and both processes involve numerous neurotransmitters, neuromodulators, and receptors of primary afferent neurons relaying pain signals from the periphery to the central nervous system (Bridges et al., 2001; Kidd and Urban, 2001). Substance P (a well-known tachykinin peptide) encoded by the preprotachykinin-A (PPT-A) gene, an important neurotransmitter and/or a neuromodulator, is synthesized in the dorsal root ganglia (DRG) and released from primary afferent neurons to convey nociceptive information and transmit pain (Cao et al., 1998; Snijdelaar et al., 2000; Tang et al., 2007).

PGE_2 is a well-known pain and proinflammatory mediator abundantly produced in inflamed tissue. PGE_2-induced nociception is mediated through its four EP receptors expressed in nociceptive DRG neurons (nociceptors) and in the spinal dorsal horn neurons (Vanegas and Schaible 2001). It causes pain by directly exciting nociceptors (Vanegas and Schaible 2001) and indirectly stimulating the release of pain-related neuropeptides including substance P and calcitonin gene-related peptide (CGRP) from nociceptors (Vasko et al. 1994; Vasko 1995, White 1996).

Activation of neuronal and glial cells in the trigeminal ganglion by IL-β leads to an elevated expression of COX-2 in these cells. Newly synthesized PGE (by COX-2) in turn activates trigeminal neurons to release CGRP. There appears to be a glia-neuron interaction in the trigeminal ganglion, demonstrating a sequential link between COX-2 and CGRP, and this interaction could be the mechanism by which COX-2 inhibitors affect migraine (Neeb et al., 2012).

Neuropathic pain is an intractable chronic pain condition caused by direct physical damage or diseases of the nervous system responsible for pain generation and transmission. It is generally manifested as spontaneous pain, hyperalgesia (exaggerated response to painful stimulation) and allodynia (painful response to innocuous stimulation). Inflammatory mediators over-produced in injured nerves play a crucial role in the initiation and maintenance of neuropathic pain. Among numerous inflammatory mediators, COX-2 and its end product PGE_2 are persistently up-regulated in infiltrating macrophages and Schwann cells in injured nerves (Ma et al., 2012). Injured nerve-derived COX-2 and PGE_2 facilitate the up-regulation of pro-inflammatory cytokine interleukin-6 (IL-6) (Ma and Quirion, 2005) and pain-related peptides substance P and CGRP in invading macrophages following partial sciatic nerve ligation (Ma and Quirion, 2006; Ma et al., 2010b). EP_4 receptor, PKA, PKC, ERK/MAPK, CREB and NFκB signaling pathways are involved in PGE_2-induced IL-6 up-regulation in DRG neurons (St-Jacques and Ma, 2011).

Injured nerve-derived COX-2 and PGE_2 also up-regulate the production of transient receptor potential vanilloid-1 (TRPV1) and brain-derived neurotrophic factor (BDNF) in DRG neurons (Ma, 2010; Ma et al., 2010a; Duarte et al., 2012). EP_1 and EP_4 receptor subtypes, PKA, ERK/MAPK and CREB signaling pathways as well as nerve growth factor (NGF) are all involved in PGE_2-induced BDNF synthesis in DRG neurons related to neuropathic pain (Duarte et al., 2012).

Perineural or intraplantar injection of a non-selective or selective COX-2 inhibitor remarkably relieved neuropathic pain (Syriatowicz et al. 1999; Ma and Eisenach 2002, 2003; Ma et al. 2010). Blocking COX-2-PGE_2-EP_1 and EP_4 signalling in injured nerves might interrupt the amplification of nociceptive responses mediated by up-regulated pain mediators in DRG neurons (St-Jacques and Ma, 2011). In clinical studies, most COX-2 inhibitors are administered orally. The amount of COX-2 inhibitors reaching injured nerves is likely not sufficient to suppress the over-production of PGE_2 (Syriatowicz et al., 1999; Ma and Eisenach, 2002). This assumption is supported by the report that perineural injections of nonselective or selective COX-2 inhibitors are able to relieve neuropathic pain in animal models. Thus, it is conceivable that COX inhibitors may be useful to treat some types of neuropathic pain via local injection, an attractive approach to secure high concentrations of COX inhibitors around injured nerves and to limit the serious cardiovascular side effects notoriously associated with systemic COX-2 inhibitors (Graham et al., 2005). With the emergence of more potent and selective COX-2 inhibitors, a new generation of nonsteroidal anti-inflammatory drugs may offer better benefits in treating certain types of neuropathic pain than the COX-2 inhibitors presently in use. This trend has been suggested by on-going phase II and III clinical trials of highly potent COX-2 inhibitors in treating neuropathic pain (Gilron and Coderre, 2007).

Prostaglandins and Thermoregulation

Prostaglandins of various kinds (E_1, E_2 and $F_{1\alpha}$) produced hyperthermia in many animal species and there seems to be no cross-species differences (Chiu and Richardson, 1985). Injections of prostaglandins E_1 or $F_{1\alpha}$ into the third ventricle of the cat caused a dose-dependent rise in body temperature (Milton and Wendlandt, 1970). PGE_2 appears to act on the anterior hypothalamus to induce fever (Coceani et al., 1989; Milton, 1989). IL-1, a potent endogenous pyrogen, acts via the synthesis of prostaglandins. In infectious diseases, IL-1 synthesis is activated and IL-1 can cross the blood-brain barrier and trigger PGE_2 synthesis.

The biosynthesis of PGE_2 can also be stimulated in cerebral microvessels by endotoxins of bacterial origin. However, injections of prostaglandins E_1, E_2 or $F_{2\alpha}$ into the hypothalamus can also elicit a hypothermic response (Artunkal et al., 1977; Artunkal and Marley, 1974). Thus, prostaglandins seem to be involved in thermoregulation.

Prostaglandins and Neural Pathogenesis

Prostaglandins are associated with several pathological conditions in the brain. The level of PGE_2 in the central nervous system is increased in various pathological conditions (Montine et al., 1999; Paoletti et al., 1998). For example, cerebral ischemia in rodents caused the up-regulation of COX-2 gene expressions and PGE_2 concentrations in the hippocampus (Ohtsuki et al., 1996; Nakayama et al., 1998). Individuals with autism spectrum disorders have elevated levels of lipid peroxidation and oxidative stress biomarkers such as 8-isoprostane-$PGF_{2\alpha}$ in the plasma (Al-Gadani et al., 2009; Mostafa et al., 2010).

The cerebrovascular actions of prostaglandins have been examined in detail (White, 1982; White and Hagen, 1982). PGE_2 and $PGF_{2\alpha}$ are the major prostaglandins in the brain and the cerebral vasculature (Gaudet et al., 1980; White and Hagen, 1982; Chemtob et al., 1990a,b). Concentrations of these prostaglandins in the blood and brain are much higher in the perinatal period than in adult life (Mitchell et al., 1978; Jones et al., 1993). Prostaglandins have been implicated in the pathogenesis of migraine (Parantainen and Vapaatalo, 1988). In addition, they seem to play a role in other pathological conditions such as cerebral vasospasm and ischemia (Watanabe et al., 1988). Furthermore, the vasodilation effect of VIP seems to be mediated by the effect of prostaglandins on dopamine release (Rotrosen and Wolkin, 1987).

Altered PGE_2 signalling due to abnormal lipid peroxidation and oxidative stress may underlie some pathologies of the nervous system. Prenatal exposure to misoprostol, a prostaglandin type E analogue, during the first and second trimester of pregnancy has been linked to a number of malformations and neurodevelopmental defects (Miller et al., 2005; Bandim et al., 2003). In summary, prostaglandins can act through specific G-protein-coupled receptors to elicit important neural functions. However, altered prostaglandin signaling due to abnormal lipid peroxidation and oxidative stress may underlie some pathologies of the nervous system. Understanding the effects and mechanisms of prostaglandin pathogenesis could link to improvements in human health.

References

Abdel-Halim, MS; Hamberg, M; Sjöquist, B; Änggård, E. Identification of prostaglandin D_2 as a major prostaglandin in homogenates of rat brain. *Prostaglandins*, 1977, 14, 663-643.

Abdel-Halim, MS; von Holst, H; Meyerson, B; Sachs, C; Änggård, E. Prostaglandin profiles in tissue and blood vessels from human brain. *J. Neurochem.*, 1980a, 34, 1331-1333.

Abdel-Halim, MS; Lunder, I; Cseh, G; Änggård, E. Prostaglandin profiles in nervous tissue and blood vessels of the brain of various animals. *Prostaglandins*, 1980b, 19, 249-258.

Abran, D; Varma, DR; Li, DY; Chemtob, S. Reduced responses of retinal vessels of the newborn pig to prostaglandins but not to thromboxane. *Can. J. Physiol. Pharmac.*, 1994, 72, 168-173.

Ajmone-Cat, MA; Iosif, RE; Ekdahl, CT; Kokaia, Z; Minghetti, L; Lindvall, O. Prostaglandin E_2 and BDNF levels in rat hippocampus are negatively correlated with status epilepticus severity, non-impact on survival of seizure-generated neurons. *Neurobiol. Disease*, 2006, 23, 23-35.

Al-Gadani, Y; El-Ansary, A; Attas, O; Al-Ayadhi, L. Metabolic biomarkers related to oxidative stress and antioxidant status in Saudi autistic children. *Clin. Biochem.*, 2009, 42, 1032-1040.

Artunkal, A; Marley, E. Hyper- and hypo-thermic effects of prostaglandin E_1 (PGE_1) and their potentiation by indomethacin in chicks. *J. Physiol. Lond*, 1974, 242, 141P-142P.

Artunkal, A; Marley, E; Stephenson, JD. Some effects of prostaglandins E_1 and E_2 and of endotoxin injected into the hypothalamus of young chicks, dissociation between endotoxin fever and the effects of prostaglandins. *Br. J. Pharmac.*, 1977, 61, 39-46.

Bandim, JM; Ventura, LO; Miller, MT; Almeida, HC; Costa, AE. Autism and Mobius sequence, an exploratory study of children in northesatern Brazil. *Arq. Neuropsiquiatr.*, 2003, 61, 181-185.

Bergstrom, S; Farnebo, LO; Fuxe, K. Effect of prostaglandin E_2 on central and peripheral catecholamine neurons. *Eur. J. Pharmac.*, 1973, 21, 362-368.

Bhattacharya, SK; Reddy, PKSP; Debnath, PK; Sanyal, AK. Potentiation of antinociceptive action of morphine by prostaglandin E_1 in albino rats. *Clin. Exp. Pharmac. Physiol.*, 1975, 2, 303-357.

Bloss, JL; Singer, GH. Neuropharmacological and behavioral evaluation of prostaglandin E_2 and 11-thio-11-deoxy prostaglandin E_2 in the mouse and rat. *Psychopharmac.*, 1978, 57, 295-302.

Brazel, CY; Nunez, JL; Yang, Z; Levison, SW. Glutamate enhances survival and proliferation of neural progenitors derived from the subventricular zone. *Neurosci.,* 2005, 131, 55-65.

Breyer, RM; Bagdassarian, CK; Myers, SA; Breyer, MD. Prostanoid receptors, subtypes and signalling. *Annu. Rev. Pharmac. Toxicol.*, 2001, 41, 661-690.

Bridges, D; Thompson, SW; Rice, AS. Mechanisms of neuropathic pain. *Br. J. Anaesth.*, 2001, 87, 12-26.

Burch, RM; Luini, A; Axelrod, J. Phospholipase A_2 and phospholipase C are activated by distinct GTP-binding proteins in response to α1-adrenergic stimulation in FRTL5 thyroid cells. *Proc. Natl. Acad. Sci. USA*, 1986a, 83, 7201-7205.

Burch, RM; Luini, A; Mais, DE; Corda, D; Vanderhock, JY; Kohn, LD; Axelrod, J. α1-adrenergic stimulation of arachidonic acid release and metabolism in a rat thyroid cell line. *J. Biol. Chem.,* 1986b, 261, 11236-11241.

Burks, SR; Wright, CL; McCarthy, MM. Exploration of prostanoid receptor subtype regulating estradiol and prostaglandin E_2 induction of spinophilin in developing preoptic area neurons. *Neurosci.,* 2007, 146, 1117-1127.

Cao, YQ; Mantyh, PW; Carlson, EJ; Gillespie, AM; Epstein, CJ; Basbaum, AI. Primary afferent tachykinins are required to experience moderate to intense pain. *Nature*, 1998, 392, 390-394.

Chemtob, S; Beharry, K; Rex, J; Varma, DR; Aranda, JV. Changes in cerebrovascular prostaglandins and thromboxane as a function of systemic blood flow. *Circ. Res.*, 1990a, 67, 674-682.

Chemtob, S; Beharry, K; Rex, J; Varma, DR; Aranda, JV. Prostaglandins determine the range of cerebral blood flow autoregulation of newborn piglets. *Stroke*, 1990b, 21, 777-784.

Chen, C; Magee, JC; Bazan, NG. Cyclooxygenase-2 regulates prostaglandin E_2 signaling in hippocampal long-term synaptic plasticity. *J. Neurophysiol.*, 2002, 87, 2851-2857.

Chiu, EKY; Richardson, JS. Behavioral and neurochemical aspects of prostaglandins in brain function. *Gen. Pharmac.*, 1985, 16, 163-175.

Chung-Davidson, Y-W; Bryan, MB; Teeter, J; Bedore, CN; Li, W. Neuroendocrine and behavioral responses to weak electric fields in adult sea lampreys *Petromyzon marinus*. *Horm. Behav.*, 2008a, 54, 34-40.

Chung-Davidson, Y-W; Rees, CB; Bryan, MB; Li, W. Neurogenic and neuroendocrine effects of goldfish pheromones. *J. Neurosci.,* 2008b, 28, 14492-14499.

Coceani, F; Bishai, I; Lees, J; Sirko, S. Prostaglandin E_2 in the pathogenesis of pyrogen fever, validation of an intermediary role. *Adv. Prost. Thromb. Leuk. Res.*, 1989, 19, 394-397.

Coleman, RA. Methods in prostanoid receptor classification. In: Benedetto, C; McDonald-Gibson, RG; Nigam, S; Slater, TF, eds. *Prostaglandins and related substances, a practical approach*. Oxford: IRL Press Ltd; 1987, pp. 267-303.

Coleman, RA; Kennedy, I; Sheldrick, RLG; Tolowinska, IY. Further evidence for the existence of three subtypes of PGE_2 sensitive EP receptors. *Br. J. Pharmac.*, 1987, 91, 407P.

Dave, KA; Platel, J-C; Huang, F; Tian, D; Stamboulian-Platel, S; Bordey, A. Prostaglandin E_2 induces glutamate release from subventricular zone astrocytes. *Neuron Glia Biol.*, 2010, 6, 201-207.

Debril, MB; Renaud, JP; Fajas, L; Auwerx, J. The pleiotropic functions of peroxisome proliferator-activated receptor gamma. *J. Mol. Med.*, 2001, 79, 30-47.

Desijaru, T. Effect of intraventricularly administered prostaglandin E_1 on the electrical activity of cerebral cortex and behaviour in the unanesthetized monkey. *Prostaglandins*, 1973, 3, 859-870.

Di Giorgi-Gerevini, V; Melchiorri, D; Battaglia, G; Ricci-Vitiani, L; Ciceroni, C; Busceti, CL; Biagioni, F; Iacovelli, L; Canudas, AM; Parati, E; DeMaria, R; Nicolett, F. Endogenous activation of metobotropic glutamate receptors supports the proliferation and survival of neural progenitor cells. *Cell Death Diff.*, 2005, 12, 1124-1133.

Duarte, PC; St-Jacques, B; Ma, W. Prostaglandin E_2 contributes to the synthesis of brain-derived neurotrophic factor in primary sensory neuron in ganglion explant cultures and in a neuropathic pain model. *Exp. Neurol.*, 2012, 234, 466-481.

Egg, D; Herold, M; Rumpl, E; Gunther, R. Prostaglandin $F_{2\alpha}$ level in human cerebrospinal fluid in normal and pathological conditions. *J. Neurol.*, 1980, 222, 239-248.

Eglen, RM; Whiting, RL. Characterization of the prostanoid receptor profile of enprostil and isomers in smooth muscle and platelets *in vitro*. *Br. J. Pharmac.*, 1989, 98, 1335-1343.

Eguchi, N; Hayashi, H; Urade, Y; Ito, S; Hayashi, O. Central action of prostaglandin E_2 and its methyl ester in the induction of hyperthermia after their systemic administration in urethane-anesthetized rats. *J. Pharmac. Exp. Ther.*, 1988, 247, 671-679.

Feldberg, W; Milton, AS. Prostaglandins and body temperature. In: Vane JR, Ferveira SH, eds. *Handbook of Experimental Pharmacology*. Berlin: Springer-Verlag; 1978, pp. 615-656.

Feldberg, W; Sherwood, SL. Behaviour of cats after intraventricular injections of eserine and DFP. *J. Physiol. Lond.*, 1954, 125, 488-500.

Feldberg, W; Sherwood, SL. Injections of bulbocapnine into the cerebral ventricles of cats. *Br. J. Pharmac.*, 1955, 10, 371-374.

Ferreira, SH; Vane, JR. Prostaglandins, their disappearance from and release into the circulation. *Nature,* 1967, 216, 868-873.

Gaudet, RJ; Alam, I; Levine, L. Accumulation of cyclooxygenase products of arachidonic acid metabolism in gerbil brain during reperfusion after bilateral common carotid artery occlusion. *J. Neurochem.*, 1980, 35, 653-658.

Gerber, JG; Payne, NA; Murphy, RC; Nies, AS. Prostacyclin produced by the pregnant uterus in the dog may act as a circulating vasodepressor substance. *J. Clin. Invest.*, 1981, 67, 632-636.

Forman, BM; Tontonoz, P; Chen, J; Brun, RP; Spiegelman, BM; Evans, RM. 15-Deoxy-$\Delta^{12,14}$-prostaglandin J_2 is a ligand for the adipocyte determination factor PPAR gamma. *Cell*, 1995, 83, 803-812.

Giles, H; Leff, P. The biology and pharmacology of PGD_2. *Prostaglandins*, 1988, 35, 277-300.

Gilmore, DP; Shaikh, AA. The effects of prostaglandin E_2 in producing sedation in the rat. *Prostaglandins*, 1972, 2, 143-151.

Gilron, I; Coderre, TJ. Emerging drugs in neuropathic pain. *Expert Opin. Emerg. Drugs*, 2007, 12, 113-126.

Graham, DJ; Campen, D; Hui, R; Spence, M; Cheetham, C; Levy, G; Shoor, S; Ray, WA. Risk of acute myocardial infarction and sudden cardiac death in patients treated with cyclo-oxygenase 2 selective and non-selective non-steroidal anti-inflammatory drugs, nested case control study. *Lancet*, 2005, 365, 475-481.

Gryglewski, RJ; Bunting, S; Moncada, S; Flower, RJ; Vane, JR. Arterial walls are protected against deposition of platelet thrombi by a substance prostaglandin X which they make from prostaglandin endoperoxides. *Prostaglandins*, 1976, 12, 685-708.

Guzmán-Marín, R; Suntsova, N; Stewart, DR; Gong, H; Szymusiak, R; McGinty, D. Sleep deprivation reduces proliferation of cells in the dentate gyrus of the hippocampus in rats. *J. Physiol.*, 2003, 549, 563-571.

Halushka, PV; Mais, DE; Mayeux, PR; Morinelli, TA. Thromboxane, prostaglandin and leukotriene receptors. *Annu. Rev. Pharmac. Toxicol.*, 1989, 10, 213-239.

Hata, AN; Breyer, RM. Pharmacology and signalling of prostaglandin receptors, multiple roles in inflammation and immune modulation. *Pharmac. Ther.*, 2004, 103, 147-166.

Hayaishi, O. Sleep-wake regulation by prostaglandins D_2 and E_2. *J. Biol. Chem.*, 1988, 263, 14593-14596.

Hayaishi, O. Prostaglandin D_2 and sleep. *Ann. NY Acad. Sci.*, 1989, 559, 374-381.

Hayaishi, O. Molecular genetic studies on sleep-wake regulation: with special emphasis on the prostaglandin D_2 system. *J. Appl. Physiol.*, 2002, 92,863-868.

Hayashi, H; Ito, S; Tanaka, T; Negishi, M; Kawabe, H; Yokohama, H; Watanabe, K; Hayaishi, O. Determination of 9α, 11β-prostaglandin F_2 by stereospecific antibody in various rat tissues. *Prostaglandins*, 1987, 33, 517-530.

Hedqvist, P. Studies on the effect of prostaglandins E_1 and E_2 on the sympathetic neurotransmitter transmission in some animal tissues. *Acta Physiol. Acand.*, 1970, 345, 1-40.

Herlong, JL; Scott, TR. Positioning prostanoids of the D and J series in the immunopathogenic scheme. *Immunol. Lett.*, 2006, 102, 121-131.

Hertting, G; Seregi, A. Formation and function of eicosanoids in the central nervous system. *Ann. NY Acad. Sci.*, 1989, 559, 85-99.

Hillier, K; Roberts, PJ; Templeton, WW. Prostaglandin and noradrenaline interactions in rat brain synaptosome. *Br. J. Pharmac.*, 1979, 66, 102P-103P.

Hillier, K; Roberts, PJ; Woolard, P. Catecholamine stimulated prostaglandin synthesis in rat brain synaptosomes. *Br. J. Pharmac.*, 1976, 58, 426P-427P.

Horton, EW; Main, IHM. Differences in the effects of prostaglandin $F_{2\alpha}$: a constituent of cerebral tissue, and prostaglandin E_1 on conscious cats and chicks. *Int. J. Neuropharmac.*, 1965, 4, 65-69.

Huang, ZL; Urade, Y; Hayaishi, O. Prostaglandins and adenosine in the regulation of sleep and wakefulness. *Curr. Opin. Pharmac.*, 2007, 7, 33-38.

Ito, S; Narumiya, S; Hayaishi, O. Prostaglandin D_2, a biochemical perspective. *Prost. Leuk. Essen. Fatty Acids*, 1989, 37, 219-234.

Ito, S; Sugama, K; Inagaki, N; Fukui, H; Giles, H; Wada, H; Hayaishi, O. Type-1 and type-2 astrocytes are distinct targets for prostaglandins D_2, E_2 and $F_{2\alpha}$. *Glia*, 1992, 6, 67-74.

Jones, SA; Adamson, SL; Bishai, I; Lees, J; Engelberts, D; Coceani, F. Eicosanoids in third ventricular cerebrospinal fluid of fetal and newborn sheep. *Am. J. Physiol. Regu. Integ. Comp. Physiol.*, 1993, 264, R135-R142.

Juan, H. Prostaglandins as modulators of pain. *Gen. Pharmac.*, 1978, 9, 403-409.

Jumblatt, MM; Paterson, CA. Prostaglandin E_2 effects on corneal endothelial cyclic adenosine monophosphate synthesis and cell shape are mediated by a receptor of the EP_2 subtype. *Invest. Ophthalmol. Vis. Sci.*, 1991, 32, 360-365.

Katura, T; Moriya, T; Nakahata, N. 15-Deoxy-$\Delta^{12,14}$-prostaglandin J_2 biphasically regulates the proliferation of mouse hippocampal neural progenitor cells by modulating the Redox state. *Mol. Pharmac.,* 2010, 77, 601-611.

Kempermann, G; Kuhn, HG; Gage, FH. More hippocampal neurons in adult mice living in an enriched environment. *Nature*, 1997, 386, 493-495.

Kempermann, G; Kuhn, HG; Gage, FH. Experience-induced neurogenesis in the senescent dentate gyrus. *J. Neurosci.*, 1998, 18, 3206-3212.

Kennedy, I; Coleman, RA; Humphrey, PPA; Levy, GP; Lumley, P. Studies on the characterization of prostanoid receptors, a proposed classification. *Prostaglandins*, 1982, 24, 667-689.

Kidd, BL; Urban, LA. Mechanisms of inflammatory pain. *Br. J. Anaesth.*, 2012, 87, 3-11.

Kontos, HA; Wei, EP; Ellis, EF; Dietrich, WD; Povlishock, JT. Prostaglandins in physiological and in certain pathological responses of the cerebral circulation. *Fedn. Proc. Fern. Am. Socs. Exp. Biol.,* 1981, 40, 2326-2330.

Kumihashi, K; Uchida, K; Miyazaki, H; Kobayashi, J; Tsushima, T; Machida, T. Acetylsalicylic acid reduces ischemia-induced proliferation of dentate cells in gerbils. *Neuroreport,* 2001, 12, 915-917.

Lazarus. M. The differential role of prostaglandin E_2 receptor EP_3 and EP_4 in regulation of fever. *Mol. Nutr. Food Res.*, 2006, 50, 451-455.

Li, DY; Varma, DR; Chatterjee, TK; Fernandez, H; Abran, D; Chemtob, S. Fewer PGE_2 and $PGF_{2\alpha}$ receptors in brain synaptosomes of newborn than of adult pigs. *J. Pharmac. Exp. Ther.*, 1993, 267, 1292-1297.

Li, DY; Varma, DR; Chemtob, S. Ontogenic increase in PGE_2 and $PGF_{2\alpha}$ receptor density in brain microvessels of pigs. *Br. J. Pharmac.,* 1994, 112, 59-64.

Li, Y-S; Wang, J-X; Jia, M-M; Liu, M; Li, X-J; Tang, H-B. Dragon's blood inhibits chronic inflammatory and neuropathic pain responses by blocking the synthesis and release of substance P in rats. *J. Pharmac. Sci.*, 2012, 118, 43-54.

Liu, J; Solway, K; Messing, RO; Sharp, FR. Increased neurogenesis in the dentate gyrus after transient global ischemia in gerbils. *J. Neurosci.,* 1998, 18, 7768-7778.

Lois, C; Alvarez-Buylla, A. Long-distance neuronal migration in the adult mammalian brain. *Sci.*, 1994, 264, 1145-1148.

Luskin, MB. Restricted proliferation and migration of postnatally generated neurons derived from the forebrain subventricular zone. *Neuron*, 1993, 11, 173-189.

Ma, W. Chronic prostaglandin E_2 treatment induces the synthesis of the pain-related peptide substance P and calcitonin gene-related peptide in cultured sensory ganglion explants. *J. Neurochem.,* 2010, 115, 363-372.

Ma, W; Chabot, JG; Vercauteren, F; Quirion, R. Injured nerve-derived $COX2/PGE_2$ contributes to the maintenance of neuropathic pain in aged rats. *Neurobiol. Aging,* 2010a, 31, 1227-1237.

Ma, W; Dumont, Y; Vercauteren, F; Quirion, R. Lipopolysaccharide induces calcitonin gene-related peptide in the RAW264.7 macrophage cell line. *Immunol.*, 2010b, 130, 399-409.

Ma, W; Eisenach, JC. Morphological and pharmacological evidence for the role of peripheral prostaglandins in the pathogenesis of neuropathic pain. *Eur. J. Neurosci.,* 2002, 15, 1037-1047.

Ma, W; Eisenach, JC. Cyclooxygenase 2 in infiltrating inflammatory cells in injured nerve is universally up-regulated following various types of nerve injury. *Neurosci.,* 2003a, 121, 691-704.

Ma, W; Quirion, R. Up-regulation of interleukin 6 induced by prostaglandin E_2 from invading macrophages following nerve injury, an *in vivo* and *in vitro* study. *J. Neurochem.,* 2005, 93, 664-673.

Ma, W; Quirion, R. Increased calcitonin gene-related peptide in neuroma and invading macrophages is involved in the up-regulation of interleukin-6 and nerve injury associated thermal hyperalgesia in a rat model of mononeuropathy. *J. Neurochem.,* 2006, 98, 180-192.

Matsumura, H; Honda, K; Choi, WS; Inoué, S; Sakai, T; Hayaishi, O. Evidence that brain prostaglandin E_2 is involved in physiological sleep-wake regulation in rats. *Proc. Natl. Acad. Sci. USA,* 1989, 86, 5666-5669.

Miller, MT; Stromland, K; Ventura, L; Johansson, M; Bandim, JM; Gillberg, C. Autism associated with conditions characterized by developmental errors in early embryogenesis, a mini review. *Int. J. Dev. Neurosci.,* 2005, 23, 201-219.

Milton, AS. Thermoregulatory actions of eicosanoids in the central nervous system with particular regard to the pathogenesis of fever. *Ann. NY Acad. Sci.,* 1989, 559, 392-410.

Milton, AS; Wendlandt, S. A possible role for prostaglandin E_1 as a modulator for temperature regulation in the central nervous system of the cat. *J. Physiol. Lond.,* 1970, 207, 76P-77P.

Minami, T; Nakano, H; Kobayashi, T; Sugimoto, Y; Ushikubi, F; Ichikawa, A; Narumiya, S; Ito, S. Characterization of EP receptor subtypes responsible for prostaglandin E_2-induced pain responses by use of EP_1 and EP_3 receptor knockout mice. *Br. J. Pharmac.,* 2001, 133, 438-444.

Mitchell, MD; Lucas, A; Etches, PC; Brant, JD; Turnbull, AC. Plasma prostaglandin levels during early neonatal life following term and preterm delivery. *Prostaglandins,* 1978, 16, 319-326.

Mo, N; Ammari, R; Dun, NJ. Prostaglandin E_1 inhibits calcium-dependent potentials in mammalian sympathetic neurons. *Brain Res.,* 1985, 334, 325-329.

Moncada, S; Ferreira, SH; Vane, JR. Bioassay of prostaglandins and biologically active substances derived from arachidonic acid. *Adv. Prost. Throm. Res.,* 1978, 5, 211-236.

Montine, TJ; Sidell, KR; Crews, BC; Markesbery, WR; Marnett, LJ; Roberts, LJ; Morrow, JD. Elevated CSF prostaglandin E_2 levels in patients with probable AD. *Neurol.,* 1999, 53, 1495-1498.

Mostafa, GA; El-Hadidi, ES; Hewedi, DH; Abdou, MM. Oxidative stress in Egyptian children with autism, relation to autoimmunity. *J. Neuroimmunol.,* 2010, 219, 114-118.

Nakayama, M; Uchimura, K; Zhu, RL; Nagayama, T; Rose, ME; Stetler, RA; Isakson, PC; Chen, J; Graham, SH. Cyclooxygenase-2 inhibition prevents delayed death of CA1 hippocampal neurons following global ischemia. *Proc. Natl. Acad. Sci. USA,* 1998, 95, 10954-10959.

Nakatomi, H; Kuriu, T; Okabe, S; Yamamoto, S; Hatano, O; Kawahara, N; Tamura, A; Kirino, T; Nakafuku, M. Regeneration of hippocampal pyramidal neurons after ischemic brain injury by recruitment of endogenous neural progenitors. *Cell,* 2002, 110, 429-441.

Narumiya, S; Ogorochi, T; Nakao, K; Hayaishi, O. Prostaglandin D_2 in rat brain, spinal cord and pituitary: basal level and regional distribution. *Life Sci.,* 1982, 31, 2093-2103.

Neeb, L; Hellen, P; Boehnke, C; Hoffmann, J; Schuh-Hofer, S; Dirnagl, U; Reuter, U. IL-1β stimulates COX-2 dependent PGE_2 synthesis and CGRP release in rat trigeminal ganglia cells. *PLoS One*, 2012, 63, e17360.

Nistico, G; Marley, E. Central effects of prostaglandins E_2; A_1 and $F_{2\alpha}$ in adult fowls. *Neuropharmac.*, 1976, 15, 737-741.

Nottebohm, F. From bird song to neurogenesis. *Sci. Am.*, 1989, 260, 74-79.

Nottebohm, F. Neuronal replacement in adulthood. *Ann. NY Acad. Sci.*, 1985, 457, 143-161.

Ogorochi, T; Narumiya, S; Mizuno, N; Yamashita, K; Miyazaki, H; Hayaishi, O. Regional distribution of prostaglandins D_2, E_2 and $F_{2\alpha}$ and related enzymes in *post-mortem* human brain. *J. Neurochem.*, 1984, 43, 71-82.

Ohtsuki, T; Kitagawa, K; Yamagata, K; Mandai, K; Mabuchi, T; Matsishita, K; Yanagihara, T; Matsumoto, M. Induction of cyclooxygenase-2 mRNA in gerbil hippocampal neurons after transient forebrain ischemia. *Brain Res.*, 1996, 736, 353-356.

Olson, AK; Eadie, BD; Ernst, C; Christie, BR. Environmental enrichment and voluntary exercise massively increase neurogenesis in the adult hippocampus via dissociable pathways. *Hippocampus*, 2006, 16, 250-260.

Paoletti, AM; Piccirilli, S; Costa, N; Rotiroti, D; Bagetta, G; Nistico, G. Systemic administration of N omega-nitro-L-arginine methyl ester and indomethacin reduces the elevation of brain PGE_2 content and prevents seizures and hippocampal damage evoked by LiCl and tacrine in rat. *Exp. Neurol.*, 1998, 149, 349-355.

Parantainen, J; Vapaatalo, H. Prostaglandins in the pathophysiology of migraine. In: Curtis-Prior PB, ed. *Prostaglandins Biology and Chemistry of Prostaglandins and Related Eicosanoids*. Edinburgh: Churchill Livingstone; 1988, pp. 386-401.

Parent, JM; Yu, TW; Leibowitz, RT; Geschwind, DH; Sloviter, RS; Lowenstein, DH. Dentate granule cell neurogenesis is increased by seizures and contributes to aberrant network reorganization in the adult hippocampus. *J. Neurosci.*, 1997, 17, 3727-3738.

Platel, JC; Dave, KA; Bordey, A. Control of neuroblast production and migration by converging GABA and glutamate signals in the postnatal forebrain. *J. Physiol.*, 2008, 586, 3739-3743.

Platel, JC; Dave, KA; Gordon, V; Lacar, B; Rubio, ME; Bordey, A. NMDA receptors activated by subventricular zone astrocytic glutamate are critical for neuroblast survival prior to entering a synaptic network. *Neuron*, 2010, 65, 859-872.

Reichman, M; Nen, W; Hokin, LE. Highly sensitive muscarinic receptors in the cerebellum are coupled to prostaglandin formation. *Biochem. Biophys. Res. Comm.*, 1987, 146, 1256-1261.

Reimann, W; Steinhauer, HB; Hedler, L; Starke, K; Hertting, G. Effect of prostaglandins D_2, E_2 and $F_{2\alpha}$ on catecholamine release from slices of rat and rabbit brain. *Eur. J. Pharmac.*, 1981, 69, 421-427.

Roberts II, LJ; Sweetman, BJ; Lewis, RA; Austen, KF; Oates, JA. Increased production of prostaglandin D_2 in patients with systemic mastocytosis. *New Engl. J. Med.*, 1980, 303, 1400-1404.

Rotrosen, J; Wolkin, A. Phospholipid and prostaglandin hypotheses of schizophrenia. In: Meltzer HY, ed. *Psychopharmacology. The Third Generation of Progress*. New York: Raven Press; 1987, pp. 759-764.

Samuelsson, B. Identification of a smooth muscle-stimulating factor in bovine brain prostaglandins and related factors. *Biochem. Biophys. Acta*, 1964, 84, 218-219.

Sandeman, R; Sandeman, D. Impoverished and enriched living conditions influence the proliferation and survival of neurons in crayfish brain. *J. Neurobiol.,* 2000, 45, 215-226.

Santoian, EC; Angerio, AD; Schneidkraut, MJ; Ramwell, PW; Kot, PA. Role of calcium in U46619 and $PGF_{2\alpha}$ pulmonary vasoconstriction in rat lungs. *Am. J. Physiol. Heart Circ. Physiol.* 1989, 257, H2001-H2005.

Sanyal, AK; Srivastava, DN; Bhattacharya, SK. The antinociceptive effect of intracerebroventricularly administered prostaglandin E_1 in the rat. *Psychopharmac.,* 1979, 60, 159-163.

Sasaki, T; Kassell, NF; Torner, JC; Maixner, W; Turner, DM. Pharmacological comparison of isolated monkey and dog cerebral arteries. *Stroke,* 1985, 16, 482-489.

Schaad, NC; Magistretti, PJ; Schorderet, M. Prostanoids and their role in cell-cell interactions in the central nervous system. *Neurochem. Int.,* 1991, 18, 303-322.

Schaad, NC; Schorderet, M; Magistretti, PJ. The accumulation of cAMP elicited by vasoactive intestinal peptide VIP is potentiated by noradrenaline, histamine, adenosine, baclofen, phorbol esters and ouabain in mouse cerebral cortical slices studies on the role of arachidonic acid metabolites and protein kinase C. *J. Neurochem.,* 1989, 53, 1941-1951.

Schaefer, A; Komlos, M; Seregi, A. Effects of biogenic amines and psychotropic drugs on endogenous prostaglandin biosynthesis in the rat brain homogenates. *Biochem. Pharmac.,* 1978, 27, 213-218.

Scotto-Lomassese, S; Strambi, C; Strambi, A; Charpin, P; Augier, R; Aouane, A; Cayre, M. Influence of environmental stimulation on neurogenesis in the adult insect brain. *J. Neurobiol.,* 2000, 45, 162-171.

Seregi, A; Hertting, G. Changes in cyclooxygenase activity and prostaglandin profiles during monoamine metabolism in rat brain homogenates. *Prost. Leuk. Med.,* 1984, 14, 113-121.

Smith, WL. The eicosanoids and their biochemical mechanisms of action. *Biochem. J.,* 1989, 259, 315-324.

Smith, WL. Prostanoid biosynthesis and mechanisms of action. *Am. J. Physiol. Renal. Physiol.,* 1992, 263, F181-F191.

Smith, WL; Marnett, LJ; DeWitt, DL. Prostaglandin and thromboxane biosynthesis. *Pharmac. Ther.,* 1991, 49, 153-179.

Smith, WL; Urade, Y; Jakobsson, P-J. Enzymes of the cyclooxygenase pathways of prostanoid biosynthesis. *Chem. Rev.,* 2011, 11110, 5821-5865.

Snijdelaar, DG; Dirksen, R; Slappendel, R; Crul, BJ. Substance P. *Eur. J. Pain,* 2000, 4, 121-135.

Sorensen, PW; Goetz, FW. Pheromonal and reproductive function of F prostaglandins and their metabolites in teleost fish. *J. Lipid Med.,* 1993, 6, 385-393.

Sorensen, PW; Hara, TJ; Stacey, NE; Goetz, FW. F prostaglandins function as potent olfactory stimulants that comprise the postovulatory female sex pheromone in goldfish. *Biol. Reprod.,* 1988, 39, 1039-1050.

Sorensen, PW; Stacey, NE; Chamberlain, KJ. Differing behavioral and endocrionological effects of two female sex pheromones on male goldfish. *Horm. Behav.,* 1989, 23, 317-322.

Stacey, NE. Roles of hormones and pheromones in fish reproductive behavior. In: Crews D, ed. *Psychobiology of reproductive behavior: an evolutionary perspective.* Englewood Cliffs: Prentice-Hall; 1987, pp. 28-60.

Stacey, NE; Peter, RE. Central action of prostaglandins in spawning behavior of female goldfish. *Physiol. Behav.,* 1979, 22, 1191-1196.

Steinhauer, H; Anhut, H; Hertting, G. Induction of prostaglandin synthesis in the mouse brain by convulsive drugs. *Naunyn-Schmiedebergs Archs. Pharmac.*, 1979, 307, R69.

St-Jacques, B; Ma, W. Role of prostaglandin E_2 in the synthesis of the proinflammatory cytokine interleukin-6 in primary sensory neurons, an *in vivo* and *in vitro* study. *J. Neurochem.,* 2011, 118, 841-854.

Suba, EA; Roth, BL. Prostaglandins activate phosphoinositide metabolism in rat aorta. *Eur. J. Pharmac.,* 1987, 136, 325-332.

Sugimoto, Y; Namba, T; Honda, A; Hayashi, Y; Negishi, M; Ichikawa, A; Narumiya, S. Cloning and expression of a cDNA for mouse prostaglandin E_2 receptor EP_3 subtype. *J. Biol. Chem.*, 1992, 267, 6463-6466.

Sun, FF; Chapman, JP; McGuire, JC. Metabolism of prostaglandin endoperoxide in animal tissues. *Prostaglandins*, 1977, 14, 1055-1074.

Syriatowicz, JP; Hu, D; Walker, JS; Tracey, DJ. Hyperalgesia due to nerve injury: role of prostaglandins. *Neurosci.*, 1999, 94, 587-594.

Tamiji, J; Crawford, DA. Prostaglandin E_2 and misoprostol induce neurite retraction in neuro-2a cells. *Biochem. Biophys. Res. Comm.*, 2010, 398, 450-456.

Tang, HB; Li, YS; Arihiro, K; Nakata, Y. Activation of the neurokinin-1 receptor by substance P triggers the release of substance P from cultured adult rat dorsal root ganglion neurons. *Mol. Pain,* 2007, 3, 42.

Templeton, WW. Prostanoid actions on transmitter release. In: Curtis-Prior PB, ed. *Prostaglandins Biology and Chemistry of Prostaglandins and Related Eicosanoids.* Edinburgh: Churchill Livingstone; 1988, pp. 402-410.

Uchida, K; Kumihashi, K; Kurosawa, S; Kobayashi, T; Itoi, K; Machida, T. Stimulatory effects of prostaglandin E_2 on neurogenesis in the dentate gyrus of the adult rat. *Zool. Sci.,* 2002, 19, 1211-1216.

Vanegas, H; Schaible, HG. Prostaglandin and cycloxygenases in the spinal cord. *Prog. Neurobiol.*, 2001, 64, 327-363.

Vasko, MR. Prostaglandin-induced neuropeptide release from spinal cord. *Prog. Brain Res.*, 1995, 104, 367-380.

Vasko, MR; Campbell, WB; Waite, KJ. Prostaglandin E_2 enhances bradykinin-stimulated release of neuropeptides from rat sensory neurons in culture. *J. Neurosci.*, 1994, 14, 4987-4997.

Vasko, MR; Crider, J; Campbell, W. Prostaglandins increase the release of substance P from cultured sensory neurons. *Soc. Neurosci. Abtr.,* 1989, 15, 471.

White, DM. Mechanism of prostaglandin E_2-induced substance P release from cultured sensory neurons. *Neurosci.,* 1996, 70, 561-565.

Walczak, R; Tontonoz, P. PPARadigms and PPARadoxes, expanding roles for PPARγ in the control of lipid metabolism. *J. Lipid. Res.*, 2002, 43, 177-186.

Watanabe, T; Asano, T; Shimizu, T; Seyama, Y; Takakura, K. Participation of lipoxygenase products from arachidonic acid in the pathogenesis of cerebral vasospasm. *J. Neurochem.,* 1988, 50, 1145-1150.

White, RP. Prostaglandins and cerebral vasospasm. In: Greenberg S, Kadowitz PJ, Burks TF, eds. *Modern Pharmacology Toxicology* Vol. 2. New York: Dekker; 1982.

White, RP; Hagen, AA. Cerebrovascular actions of prostaglandins. *Pharmac. Ther.*, 1982, 18, 313-331.

Wolfe, LS. Arachidonic acid metabolites and the nervous system, and appraisal of the present situation. In: Curtis-Prior PB, ed. *Prostaglandins Biology and Chemistry of Prostaglandins and Related Eicosanoids*. Edinburgh: Churchill Livingstone; 1988, pp. 411-421.

Wolfe, LS; Rostworowski, K; Pappius, HM. The endogenous biosynthesis of prostaglandins by brain tissue *in vitro. Can. J. Biochem.*, 1976, 54, 629-640.

Yamamoto, S. Characterization of enzymes in prostanoid synthesis. In: Curtis-Prior PB, ed. *Prostaglandins Biology and Chemistry of Prostaglandins and Related Eicosanoids*. Edinburgh: Churchill Livingstone; 1988, pp. 37-45.

Zhu, P; Genc, A; Zhang, X; Zhang, J; Bazan, NG; Chen, C. Heterogeneous expression and regulation of hippocampal prostaglandin E_2 receptors. *J. Neurosci .Res.*, 2005, 81, 817-826.

In: Advances in Medicine and Biology. Volume 69   ISBN: 978-1-62808-088-9
Editor: Leon V. Berhardt   © 2013 Nova Science Publishers, Inc.

Chapter II

Prostaglandin E₁: Action Mechanism, Biological Effects and its Clinical Significance in Improving Peripheral Arterial Blood Flow

Mario González Gay and Amer Zanabili Al-Sibbai
Department of Angiology and Vascular Surgery, Hospital
Universitario Central de Asturias, Oviedo, Spain

Abstract

Prostaglandin E_1 (PGE_1) is a hormonal compound that shares with other prostaglandin series its origin as a metabolite of polyunsaturated fatty acids, constituent of cell membrane phospholipids, and the diversity of its autocrine and paracrine biological activities. This broad profile of actions ranges from inhibition of the chemiotaxis and the activation of white cells, to profibrinolytic effect and reduction of hematic viscosity. Amongst the pharmacodynamic properties of PGE_1, improvement of the peripheral circulation is probably the most significant of its biological effects. The action is induced by a potent peripheral vasodilation and the inhibition of platelet aggregation and adhesion, mediated by cyclic adenosine-monohophosphate (cAMP).

These activities, once it is liberated to the circulation, are mostly loco-regional due to its fast enzyme inactivation, which reaches up to 90% after first lung passage and a half life in plasma of less than two minutes. The chemical stability and hydrophobicity can be improved significantly by complexing PGE_1 to other molecules, like α-ciclodextrin, making it suitable for exogenous administration and therapeutic use.

The vasoactive properties of PGE_1 make it a valuable tool for the treatment of peripheral arterial disease and critical limb ischemia in particular, amongst other medical applications. In a clinical situation in which perfusion has been reduced to a point that viability of the limb is dramatically endangered, PGE_1 is the pharmacological treatment of choice in many occasions. This takes place when surgical and endovascular solutions are not an option, failed or as an adjuvant treatment of those therapies, due to its capacity to improve macro and micro circulation. Although traditionally this anti-ischemic action was explained by the combined direct vasodilation and inhibition of platelet function, recent experimental findings suggest that more factors may contribute to its clinical efficacy. This includes anti-inflammatory effects, inhibition of expression of adhesion molecules and generation and release of growth factors, suggesting an improvement in endothelial function and a decrease of vascular cell activation, which could explain the long-term benefits on PGE_1. Its clinical use covers a broad range of ischemic related disorders including peripheral arterial occlusive disease, Reynaud syndrome, scleroderma, Lupus, Buerger's disease, ergotism, atheroembolic disease, hypertensive ulcers, etc. Because of its rapid inactivation during lung passage, PGE_1 has to be administered either intra-arterial or in large doses intravenous, in order to treat peripheral arterial disease. While intra-arterial applications had been recommended initially, the high rate of secondary effects and complications make intravenous infusions the preferred application route at present. In this chapter we will explore the biochemistry, physiological role and therapeutic potential of the PGE_1, along with the latest advances on its use in the treatment of clinical entities involving peripheral ischemia.

Introduction

Prostaglandin E_1 (PGE_1), like the rest of the prostaglandin series, is a 20 carbon polyunsaturated fatty acid whose major precursor in most animals is the arachidonic acid. They are a heterogeneous group of hormones, constituent of cell membrane phospholipids, with a diverse range of biological activities.

As messenger molecules their action takes place locally, either in the same cell that secretes it or in nearby cells (autocrin and paracrin signaling) due to the rapid inactivation by enzymes, and their production can be located all throughout the body and not in a specific organ or tissue. This explains the powerful effect of prostaglandins in a variety of biological systems apparently none related one to another. The presence of a smooth muscle stimulating factor in sperm and in extracts of the accessory genital glands of man and certain animals was reported by Goldblatt and von Vouler as early as 1933 [1, 2]. Nevertheless, and partly due to the outbreak of World War II, it wouldn't be until 1957 that Bergström and Sjövall were able to isolate small amounts of two crystalline compounds from the lipid extracts stored by von Vouler since before the war [3]. These first prostaglandins, as they were named according to their origin, were PGE_1 and PGF_1. By 1962 their chemical structure had been determined, leading the way to demonstrate that prostaglandins occur in many other tissues outside the male reproductive organs. Prostaglandins are released from mammalian tissues in response to mechanical, physiological and pathological stimuli, such as hormonal, neural and inflammatory. When tested, the amount of prostaglandins released under stimulation was much greater than that released in the absence of stimulus. This indicated that prostaglandins are not preformed but synthesized when given the appropriate stimulus [4]. The ability to synthesize prostaglandin analogues and the increasing number of free samples available for research was the base for an exponentially escalating number of studies and publications based on these compounds in the following years, establishing the bases for the research this and other prostaglandins, their physiological role and the therapeutic potential in the ensuing decades. Karl Bergström, together with Samuelsson and Vane, would receive the Nobel Prize in 1982 for their research on this field.

Biochemistry and Biological Effects

All prostaglandins of the E type contain the characteristic 11α- hydroxy and 9-keto groups on a five membered ring, common to other prostaglandins. The chemical formula of PGE$_1$ was determined to be C$_{20}$H$_{34}$O$_5$ [Figure 1], with the characteristic five carbons structure. It is an oxygenated metabolite that originates from the dihomo-γ-linoleic acid, an analogue of arachidonic acid, via a membrane bound enzyme that transforms the prostaglandin endoperoxide PGE$_1$.

The first study on the cardiovascular effects of prostaglandins in humans took place shortly after their isolation, in 1959, at the Karolinska Institute of Stockholm.

When administered via continuous intra-arterial infusion into the left brachial artery, PGE$_1$ caused a fall in blood pressure and a raise in the heart rate, as well as the increase in the blood flow on the forearm [5, 6, 7]. These observations would later lead the way to a new line of therapy for peripheral vascular disease.

In 1966 Kloeze demonstrated that PGE$_1$ was able to suppress the platelet activation process, therefore effectively inhibiting platelet aggregation [8]. It was later discovered that PGE$_1$ not only inhibits the release of platelet factor 4 and β-thromboglobulin, but also the synthesis of leucotrienes and aggregation-promoting thromboxane [9, 10]. Moreover, it is also able to regulate the inhibition of neutrophil function, suppressing the chemiotaxis and the activation of white cells [11].

These effects of PGE$_1$ depend on the molecule binding to a membrane surface receptor of certain cells, like platelets, neutrophiles and smooth cells that, once activated, increases the cyclic adenosine-monophosphate (cAMP) by modulating the enzyme adenylcyclase. The activation of this mechanism, common to Prostacyclin (PGI$_2$), leads to the rise in the intracellular levels of cAMP, which will then work as a second messenger, inhibiting cell activation [12], and also resulting in a decrease of intracellular non-bound calcium through the regulation of transmembrane calcium ion flux. By counteracting any increase in cytosolic calcium levels that would result from thromboxane A2 (TXA$_2$) binding, the activation of platelets is also inhibited, subsequently preventing aggregation. In endothelial cells, the rise in cAMP activates protein kinase A (PKA). PKA then continues the cascade by phosphorylating and inhibiting myosin light-chain kinase, which leads to smooth muscle relaxation and vasodilation.

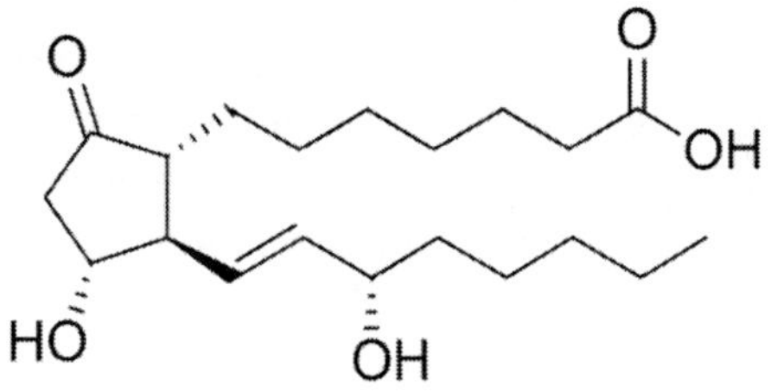

Figure 1. Chemical formula of PGE$_1$: 7-[(1R,3R)-3-hydroxy-2-[(1E,3S)-3-hydroxyoct-1-en-1-yl]-5-oxocyclopentyl]heptanoic acid.

The significant vasodilatory activity of PGE_1 is not only caused by a direct effect on the blood vessel musculature [13], but also through the antagonization of the vasoconstrictor effect of leucotriene D_4 [14]. This subsequent increase in the arterial diameter, with a maximum dilatation of the outflow tract, is followed by a corresponding reduction in peripheral resistance and a measurable rise in transcutaneous oxygen pressure, a direct indicator of capillary blood flow [15].

Other pharmacological effects of PGE_1 are the enhancement of fibrinolytic activity [16], the inhibition of the proliferation of the smooth muscle cells of the media [17], reduction of endothelial permeability and the hematic viscosity, and the stimulation of formation and growth of collateral circulation. Summarizing, all these actions account for a modulation of coagulation and fibrinolysis, anti-inflammatory effects, and improvement of regional perfusion.

Although traditionally the anti-ischemic action was explained by the combined direct vasodilatation and inhibition of platelet function, there are some long term beneficial effects of PGE_1, extending considerably beyond the time of infusion from several weeks up to a few months, which cannot be explained by the poor stability of the molecule and its short half-life, of less than a minute. This can be partially related to the incidence of biologically active metabolites, like PGE_0, with a longer period of action and comparable effects to those of PGE_1, although recent experimental findings may suggest that more factors may contribute to its clinical efficacy than those already mentioned, as other vasodilators and antiplatelet agents mostly fail to produce sustained clinical benefits [18, 19]. Likewise, any direct antiatherogenic effect would conceivable require a much longer time course than that applied during the standard treatment.

Some studies have suggested a hypolipidemic action of PGE_1, which presumably is based on a complex interaction of specific PGE_1-receptors of the liver with the LDL-apo-B,E-receptors resulting in the upregulation of the latter binding sites and thereby an increased uptake of plasma cholesterol [20]. It is also able to reduce the cholesterol content in the arterial wall, decreasing the vascular wall foam cells or diminishing lipid content per foam cell [21].

Oxidative stress and inflammation play critical roles in endothelial dysfunction. Increasing attention has now been paid to the anti-oxidant activity, anti-inflammation activity and cytoprotective action of PGE_1. Taking advantage of modern techniques of molecular biology it has been possible to enlarge the pharmacological profile of PGE_1, although some of the new effects have only been observed experimentally.

These include inhibition of expression of adhesion receptors on vascular cells (E-selectin, ICAM-1 and VCAM-1), considered to play a role in the pathogenesis of atherosclerosis and the subject of intense current investigation. Further inhibitory actions affect the endothelial release of hepatocyte growth factor, possibly preventing D-glucose mediated endothelial damage, which would be responsible in part of the improvement found in diabetics. PGE_1 has also been found to inhibit the release of inflammatory cytokines (TNFα, MCP-1) and matrix components, and to down-regulate the generation and release of growth factors, like CYR61 and CTGF [22-25].

Other studies have shown the efficacy of PGE_1 in protecting endothelial cells from oxidative injury, suppressing the production of lipid peroxides such as MDA and restoring the activity of endogenous antioxidants, while inhibiting cell apoptosis [26].

Additionally, it has been suggested that some of these changes take place at transcriptional level, both in smooth muscle vascular cells and fibroblasts. This implies that PGE$_1$ is able to modify genes which are known to be relevant for cell proliferation, migration and matrix synthesis [22], contributing to tissue preservation in lower limb ischemia.

All these actions attributed to PGE$_1$ account for a global decrease of vascular cell activation and a significant effect on endothelial protection, which ultimately would reduce the progression of atherosclerosis. Which of these factors and to which extent contribute to the overall long term efficacy of PGE$_1$ in peripheral artery disease still has to be determined, although it is now generally accepted that the sustained benefits of its treatment are the result of a complex mechanism of interactions that extends beyond the original antiaggregation/ vasodilation dual effect [Table 1].

Clinical Applications of Prostaglandin E$_1$

The potential clinical use of PGE$_1$ made it the focus of important therapeutic research soon after its discovery, although natural occurring prostaglandins faced a number of drawbacks that hindered their clinical application.

First of all, its rapid metabolism conditions any oral activity and a short duration of action when given parenterally. Second, its administration is accompanied by numerous side effects, the result of its action on multiple systems while originally intended for local signaling.

And last, a short term life due to its inherent chemical instability. To address these problems, prostaglandin analogues were researched and developed (Misoprostol, Gemeprost, Alprostadil alfadex, Limaprost alfadex...), opening the way for a new series of pharmacological treatments in different medical disciplines.

PGE$_1$ was discovered to inhibit gastric acid secretion from the parietal cells by Robert et al in 1967 [27]. It also exerts a cytoprotective effect, which makes PGE$_1$ analogues a viable oral therapy to prevent peptic ulcers. Misoprostol (15-deoxy-16-hidroxy-16-methyl PGE$_1$) is a synthetic PGE$_1$ analogue, originally developed for the prevention and treatment of peptic ulcers [28].

Table 1. Pharmacologic effects of prostaglandin E$_1$

- Inhibition of platelet activation (↓aggregation and adhesion)
- Inhibition of chemiotaxis and activation of white cells (↓ inflammation)
- Inhibition of the endothelial permeability and vasoconstrictive activity of thromboxane A2 , leukotrienes, serotonine and endothelin (↑ vasodilation)
- Inhibition of the proliferation of smooth cells of the media ⎫
- Inhibition of matrix synthesis |
- Reduction of lipid content of the arterial wall   ⎬ Endothelial protection
- Anti-oxidant endothelial activity |
- Inhibition of the expression of adhesion molecules   ⎭
- Profibrinolytic effect
- Reduction of hematic viscosity
- Stimulation of formation and growth of collateral circulation

Later, it became an important drug in obstetrics and gynecology due to its ability to induce uterus contraction and cervical priming, which probed useful in medical abortion, induction of labor and control of postpartum hemorrhage [29].

A different clinical use of PGE_1 is based on its ability to interfere with the normal closure of ductus arteriosus, which normally closes soon after birth. PGE_1 has been found useful in certain cases of ductal dependent congenital malformations (transposition of the great arteries, pulmonary atresia, pulmonary artery stenosis…) by keeping the ductus open for a few days and allowing for corrective surgery to be performed with some delay, reducing the danger to the newborn baby.

On the other hand, the closure of a ductus that remains open can be supported by the administration of cyclooxygenase inhibitors like aspirin or indomethacin, which inhibit the local prostaglandin synthesis [30].

PGE_1 has also been used for the treatment of erectile dysfunction, by injection directly into the *corpus cavernosum* or through the use of urethral suppositories [31].

Prostaglandin E_1 in Peripheral Arterial Disease

Peripheral arterial disease is a chronic pathology caused by atherosclerosis that targets any artery outside the heart, primarily in the lower extremities, although carotid arteries are frequently affected.

The clinical classification [Table 2] of the severity of this disease is based on symptoms regarding exercise limitation and lesions, and is referred to as the Fontaine Classification, introduced by René Fontaine in 1954 [32].

Disease prevalence based on objective testing has been evaluated in several epidemiologic studies, remaining in the range of 3% to 10% of the population, and increasing to 15% to 20% in people over 70 years old [33, 34, 35].

Most of the patients who present intermittent claudication as the main clinical symptom are classified as Stage II by the Fontaine classification. Intermittent claudication is caused by inadequate blood supply to muscles stressed by exercise, responsible for the common presentation symptoms of pain, cramping, numbness or weakness in certain muscles that develops during exercise and is relieved after a short rest.

The distance a person can walk before the pain develops varies in relation to the extent and severity of the arterial occlusion.

The results of follow-up studies have demonstrate that a number of patients affected by these symptoms will suffer a progressive deterioration of their clinical condition, with 10-20% experiencing severe claudication and 5-10% developing critical limb ischemia [36].

Table 2. Classification of peripheral arterial disease: Fontaine´s Stages

Grade I	Asymptomatic. Detectable by ankle-arm index <0.9	
Grade IIa	Intermittent claudication not limiting the patient´s life style	
Grade IIb	Intermittent claudication limiting for the patient	
Grade III	Pain or paresthesias at rest	} Critical ischemia
Grade IV	Established gangrene. Trophic lesions	

The five year cumulative incidence of amputation is low (1%), but intermittent claudication is an indirect sign of generalized atherosclerosis and therefore an indicator associated with increased risk of premature death [37].

A) Prostaglandin E$_1$ in Intermittent Claudication

Most patients suffering stable intermittent claudication are treated conservatively, and will not require a surgical intervention [38, 39].

There are two main targets for the conservative therapy: a) to delay the progression of atherosclerosis by controlling risk factors, like tobacco, blood pressure, diabetes, cholesterol, etc., and b) to compensate the arterial insufficiency, therefore improving the symptoms, exercise performance and the functional state of the patient.

Although it was shown that training through exercise is an effective treatment to improve the physical activity limited by claudication [40], the need for consistency in a long term basis and the concomitant diseases (e.g. cardiorespiratory insufficiency) are the reason that one third of this patients are not considered suitable candidates, and another third lack the capability or motivation for prolonged walking training. As a consequence, only 30% of these patients would finally benefit from exercise training [41]. In this context, the importance of pharmacological treatment makes PGE$_1$ a valuable asset, considering most of the therapies available focus on avoiding the progression of the disease (the base of conservative medical treatment) and very few on actually improving patient´s symptoms.

Several clinical trials [42, 43] have analyzed the effects of PGE$_1$ versus placebo in patients suffering Fontaine´s Stage IIb intermittent claudication (under 100-200 meters), both with intravenous and intra-arterial administration. They all reported a substantial improvement both in free of pain walking distance and maximum walking distance. Moreover, a significantly better long-term effect was observed with PGE$_1$ up to 6 months after the end of therapy, results that are consistent with the multiple biological effects of the molecule previously analyzed [44, 45, 46].

The Diehm trial evaluated the efficacy and security of an outpatient regimen with PGE$_1$ over 8 weeks. At the end of the treatment period the walking distance had improved 101% versus 60% of placebo, with good tolerance and a rate of adverse drug reactions of 12% [46]. Belcaro et al compared efficacy and costs of two different PGE$_1$ regimens (short-term and long-term protocols, or STP and LTP) combined with exercise, differing in the number of doses per week (five doses a week for the first two weeks, and two doses a week the four following weeks in the LTP, and two doses the weeks 0, 4, 8 and 12 in the STP). After 20 weeks of treatment the increase in walking distance was 351% in the STP and 242% in the LTP [47]. These results confirmed that with the STP less time is spent in infusion and more can be spent in the exercise program, reducing costs and, speeding up rehabilitation and expanding the number of non specialized units to follow the protocol.

Several trials [43, 48, 49] also studied the repercussion of Alprostadil Alfadex in terms of quality of life and walking distance performance in claudicant patients. A significant improvement was observed in several items: outings, personal relationships, bodily pain score and physical function. All these observations allow us to consider the treatment with PGE$_1$ a valuable therapy in patients with intermittent claudication and as a complement of physical training, in particular for those with severe walking impairment or unable to perform exercise.

B) Prostaglandin E_1 in Critical Limb Ischemia

Critical limb ischemia (CLI) is a manifestation of peripheral arterial disease that describes patients with typical chronic ischemic rest pain or patients with ischemic skin lesions, either ulcers or gangrene in one or both legs attributable to objectively proven arterial occlusive disease. The term CLI should only be used in relation to patients with chronic ischemic disease, defined as the presence of symptoms for more than 2 weeks. Left untreated, the complications will result in amputation of the affected limb.

The diagnosis of CLI should be confirmed by the ankle-brachial index, toe systolic pressure or transcutaneous oxygen tension. Ischemic rest pain most commonly occurs below an ankle pressure of 50 mmHg or a toe pressure less than 30 mmHg. For patients with ulcers or gangrene, the presence of CLI is suggested by an ankle pressure less than 70 mmHg or a toe systolic pressure less than 50 mmHg. The only reliable large prospective population studies on the incidence of CLI showed a figure of 220 new cases every year per million population [50] and it was estimated there will be approximately between 500 and 1000 new cases of CLI every year in a European or North American population of 1 million [51]. Observational studies of patients with CLI who are not candidates for revascularization suggest that a year after the onset of CLI, only about half the patients will be alive without a major amputation, although some of these may still have rest pain, gangrene or ulcers, approximately 25% will have died and 25% will have required a major amputation. The diagnosis of CLI thus predicts a poor prognosis for life and limb.

The main goals in the treatment of CLI are to relieve ischemic pain, heal ischemic ulcers, prevent limb loss, improve patient function and quality of life and prolong survival. A primary outcome would be amputation free survival. The first choice of treatment for CLI is revascularization, by reconstructive surgery or by percutaneous transluminal angioplasty or by hybrid techniques. Nevertheless, in spite of the advent of new endovascular revascularization techniques, there are still a significant number of patients unable to benefit from surgery procedures, either due to the nature of the vascular lesion or to the general debility of the patient. In other cases, revascularization alone is unable to warrant limb salvage. Thus, there is a population in which the need for medical treatment, either in isolation or as an adjunct to surgical intervention should be assessed.

Since the 70's, PGE_1 has been used worldwide as the treatment of last resort for the most serious cases of critical limb ischemia. Because of variations in the route of administration, in dosage and duration of therapy, the clinical outcome sometimes differed between studies. The first results with intra-arterial PGE_1 treatment were very encouraging, taking into account the fact that these patients did not have the possibility of revascularization, with limb amputation as the natural clinical option. Under continuous PGE_1 infusion (24 hours per day), a regression from Fontaine stage III/IV to stage IIb (claudication) was seen in 47% of non-diabetic patients with arteriosclerosis and 30% of diabetic patients with atherosclerosis [52]. Other studies reported good results with intra-arterial treatment, resulting in a significant improvement of ulcer healing, pain control and amputation rate [53, 54].

During the 80's and 90's several clinical trials studied the benefits of intravenous administration on patients with CLI. An intermittent intravenous therapy with PGE_1 was compared to placebo over a three week s period in patients suffering pain at rest. The pain decreased significantly by 67% in those treated with PGE_1 in comparison with only 8% of placebo, while 36% remitted to stage IIb compared with just 4% in the placebo group [55].

Tru☐bestein et al performed a multicenter controlled trial in patients with ischemic ulcers and/or necroses. Since the investigator refused placebo as control medication, pentoxifylline, which is registered for the treatment of intermittent claudication, was selected as a reference agent. 82% in the PGE$_1$ group showed complete or partial ulcer healing; this occurred in only 51% in the pentoxifylline group [56]. Similar results were described in diabetic patients with critical limb ischemia, with significant improvement with respect to ulcer healing, partial reduction of pain (39%) and total disappearance of pain (42%). Only 19% of the patients studied did not report benefits regarding pain reduction [57].

The long-term beneficial effects of PGE$_1$ previously reported in patients treated for intermittent claudication was also observed in more advanced stages of the disease, confirming the long-lasting clinical efficacy of the therapy in CLI. In the two trials previously mentioned, studying the effects of intravenous treatment in these patients, 6 months after the end of the treatment only 11-17% of the patients required amputation or additional surgical revascularization, compared with 34% of the patients treated with pentoxifylline or 27% of those treated with placebo, depending on the study.

In 2004, Creutzig et al published a meta-analysis evaluating the efficacy of Alprostadil in patients classified as Fountain's stage III or IV and no further possibility of revascularization [58]. Seven randomized clinical trials and 643 patients were included, reporting a significant response (ulcer healing and/or pain reduction) comparing PGE$_1$ therapy with placebo: 47.8% vs. 25.2%, respectively. A significant difference was also observed in favor of PGE$_1$ regarding the combined endpoint 'major amputation or death' after 6-month follow-up (22.6% for PGE$_1$ vs. 36.2% for placebo).

In a clinical situation in which perfusion has been reduced to a point that viability of the limb is dramatically endangered, PGE$_1$ is the pharmacological treatment of choice in many occasions. The introduction of this therapy obtained dramatic results regarding limb salvage, taking into account that PGE$_1$ often represents the last chance before amputation when the patient is not eligible for other therapies.

Prostaglandin E$_1$ in Non Atherosclerotic Ischemic Disorders

Although PGE$_1$ has widely been used for the treatment of advanced stages of peripheral arterial disease, there are other ischemic pathologies that can benefit from its pharmacological properties.

Raynaud's phenomenon (RP) is the transient digital ischemia that occurs upon exposure to cold temperature or emotional distress, the result of vasoconstriction of the digital arteries, precapillary arterioles, and cutaneous arteriovenous shunts, and that most commonly affects the fingers. Secondary RP, which is associated with various autoimmune and connective tissue diseases, like Lupus or scleroderma, involves both functional alterations and structural vascular abnormalities, and thus often results in additional complications, such as digital ulcerations that may eventually lead to amputation and increased morbidity [59].

It often does not require medical therapy, but in some cases with severe symptoms pharmacologic management is necessary.

Although PGE_1 has shown efficacy in the treatment of RP and scleroderma, reducing the frequency and severity of the attacks [60], these results have not been consistent in all the studies. A comparison between Iloprost (a stable prostacyclin analogue) and alprostadil [61] reported benefits with both treatments without significant differences in either clinical efficacy or circulating markers. However, ease of handling and the lower price favoured alprostadil. A different study suggest that alprostadil is an efficacious and well-tolerated treatment in most patients with critical ischemia secondary to RP. Iloprost proved to be still effective in those cases refractory to alprostadil, but it seemed to be somewhat less well tolerated [62]. However, in an older double-blind, placebo-controlled study enrolling patients with primary RP or RP secondary to systemic sclerosis, intravenous alprostadil was no more effective than placebo [63].

In brief, Iloprost has been more widely used and studied for the treatment of RP, being able to induce a long-lasting clinical response (up to 8 weeks) while also reducing the frequency and severity of the attacks [64]. Nevertheless, it is less stable than PGE_1, requires buffering to an alkaline pH, has a critical dose rate and its secondary effects (headache, nausea, vomiting, diarrhea...) can condition its use. Alprostadil is easier to administer, and is indicated in RP acute attacks with severe vascular compromise (ulcer and/or digital necrosis), a situation that requires hospitalization and allows for treatment monitoring.

Raynaud phenomenon has also been described with such diverse diseases as systemic lupus erythematosus and other disorders not classified as autoimmune, including frostbite, vibration injury, polyvinyl chloride exposure, and cryoglobulinemia, in which treatment with intravenous PGE_1 can also be beneficial.

Peripheral vascular ischemia secondary to ergotism is a rather uncommon condition secondary to ergotamine toxicity, usually related to chronic administration for migraine headaches. The effect of ergot alkaloids has also been known and used in obstetrics for over 400 years. They are derived from *Claviceps purpurea* fungus that grows upon grain, particularly rye, and ingestion of contaminated grain can cause intense vasoconstriction and even grangrene, a condition that during the Middle Ages was named 'St. Anthonys Fire' [65]. Despite its rare and sporadic presentation, the disorder potentially threatens limb loss and occasionally the life of the patient, taking in consideration its cardiovascular, gastrointestinal and neurological secondary effects (convulsions, delirium, nausea, vomiting, gangrene, vertigo...). Intravenous infusion with PGE_1 or PGI_2 analogues can also be considered the treatment of choice for this condition, together with the withdrawal of drugs containing ergot alkaloids, producing both vasodilation and platelet aggregation and reverting the symptoms in a few days, depending on the severity of the ischemic episode [66].

PGE_1 can also be successfully used for the treatment of another ischemic disorder, the Buerger's Disease or *thromboangiitis obliterans*. It is a peripheral arterial occlusive disease, which mainly affects the upper and lower limbs in young smokers, and while its etiology remains unknown, there is a close relationship between tobacco use and this condition. Therefore smoking cessation is the key to the correct treatment. Considering unsatisfactory results following surgical revascularization and sympathectomy in Buerger's disease [67], the use of PGE_1 and PGI_2 analogues can be considered the first-line treatment, together with a total abstinence from smoking [68, 69].

It has been used with excellent results for the treatment of hypertensive ischemic ulcers, also named Martorell's ulcers after the first clinician to describe them in 1945. These lesions, more common in women, characteristically affect the lower limbs and are accompanied by severe pain and lack of response to topical treatment. Lumbar sympathectomy was reported to improve pain control and injury healing but ulcer recidivation showed up in a high percentage, while the therapy with PGE$_1$ has shown immediate pain control and the absence of ulcer recidivation [70, 71].

Other clinical applications of prostaglandins in peripheral ischemic disorders cover atheroembolic events with no possibility of surgical revascularization [72], acute limb ischemia secondary to blunt arterial trauma [73] and any other ischemic event that due to the nature of its etiology cannot benefit from interventional treatment but nevertheless endangers the viability of the limb.

Route of Administration, Dose and Side Effects

The question about the best route of administration (intra-arterial vs. intravenous) was the subject of important controversy, given the difficult and uncomfortable handling of arterial puncture and its possible side effects, which restricted its use in practice. The intense metabolic elimination in the lungs inactivates from 60to 90% of PGE$_1$ in its first passage, responsible for a half-life of approximately 30 seconds.

As a result of this biotransformation it is possible to detect in plasma 13,14-dihydro-PGE$_1$ (also known as PGE$_0$) and 13,14-dihydro-15-keto PGE$_1$ (15-keto-PGE$_0$). With such short plasma half life it was not estrange that intra-arterial administration was clearly favored in the clinical practice during the early years of its commercialization.

Since then, several studies demonstrated that while both intra-arterial and intravenous administration afforded an equivalent improvement on clinical symptoms, intravenous perfusion was superior to intra-arterial administration regarding safety and tolerability [74, 75, 76].

There are several reasons that could explain these results: As it has been previously mentioned, the effect of PGE$_1$ does not depend entirely on arterial and arteriolar vasodilation, its benefits extending beyond the period of administration, and at least one metabolite of PGE$_1$ is pharmacologically active for longer periods, the PGE$_0$.

The dosage used for the treatment of peripheral ischemic disorders ranges from 40 µg /12 hours to 60 µg/24 hours, administered in intravenous perfusion and dissolved in 50-250 ml of physiological saline solution, during a 2-3 hours period.

The standard length of a treatment cycle is 3 weeks, which could be extended after re-evaluation of the therapeutic response. It requires strict medical control, either as part of an in-patient hospital therapy or at an outpatient facility under clinical supervision and monitoring. The safety and efficacy of the outpatient administration of PGE$_1$ in short term regimens for the treatment of intermittent claudication has been the subject of different trials [42, 77], indicating a cost effective improvement of walking distance.

This therapy is contraindicated in patients suffering from heart failure, second and third degree heart block, angina and acute myocardial infarction. The Intravenous administration can be frequently accompanied of erythema and edema in the vein being infused, although these local symptoms disappear if the dose is reduced or after suspension of the treatment. More rare side effects are headache, nausea, vomiting, hypotension and pulmonary edema.

Conclusion

Thanks to the effects of PGE_1 in different biological systems, it has found its place as the therapy for a number of medical conditions, although may be it is in the treatment of peripheral ischemic disorders were it has achieved the most important contribution. In those patients in which the evolution of their ischemia compromises the viability of the extremity, and when all surgical options have been ruled out or previously attempted without success, the pharmacological therapy with intravenous PGE_1 can be the only suitable treatment, sometimes with dramatic results.

Although the introduction of PGE_1 in the therapy of peripheral vascular disease was initially based on its vasodilatory effect and inhibitory action on platelet aggregation, it was later understood that the long-term benefit observed after the treatment involved a number of different mechanisms, some of which we are just beginning to understand. The complex interactions we have overviewed in previous pages underline a significant effect regarding endothelial protection, stabilizing the arterial wall while regulating inflammatory and smooth muscle cells, oxidative radicals and wall cholesterol. This is achieved through the control of expression and formation of adhesion molecules, inflammatory cytokines, matrix components and growth factors. In brief, PGE_1 not only facilitates perfusion to the ischemic limb, but also performs a beneficial effect on the arterial wall by reducing the damage originated by atherosclerotic disease.

References

[1]   Goldblatt, M. W. *Chemistry and Industry* 1933;52:1056-7.
[2]   Von Euler, U. S. *Arch. Exptl. Pathol. Pharmakol.* 1934;175:8.
[3]   Bergström, S., Sjövall, J. The isolation of prostaglandin. *Acta Chem. Scand.* 1957; 11:1086-90.
[4]   Piper, P. J. Distribution and metabolism. In: *The Prostaglandins. Pharmacological and Therapeutic Advances.* Ed. by Cuthbert, M. F., pp. 125-50. William Heinemann, London, 1973.
[5]   Bergström, S., et al. Observations on the effects of infusion of prostaglandin E in man. *Acta Physiol. Scand.* 1959;45:145-51.
[6]   Carlson, L. A. Metabolic and cardio-vascular effects in vivo of prostaglandins. In: *Prostaglandins, Proc. 2nd Novel Symp.*, Stockholm, June 1966, ed. by S. Bergstrom and B. Samuelsson, pp. 123-32, Almquvist and Wiksell, Stockholm; Interscience, New York, 1967.
[7]   Bevegård, S., Oro, L. Effect of prostaglandin E_1 on forearm blood flow. *Scand. J. clin. Lab. Invest.* 1969;23:347-53.
[8]   Mustard, J. F., et al. Prostaglandins and platelets. *Ann. Rev. Med.* 1980; 31:89-96.
[9]   Ham, E. A., et al. Inhibition by prostaglandins of leukotriene B4 release from activated neutrophils. *Proc. Natl. Acad. Sci. US* 1983 Jul.;80(14): 4349-53.
[10] Schrör, K., Hecker, G. Potent inhibition of superoxide anion generation by PGE_1 and the PGE_1 analogue OP-1206 in human PMN's--unrelated to its antiplatelet PGI2-like activity. *Vasa Suppl.* 1987;17:11-6.

[11] Hecker, G., et al. Cytotoxic enzyme release and oxygen centered radical formation in human neutrophils are selectively inhibited by E-type prostaglandins but not by PGI2. *Naunyn Schmiedebergs Arch. Pharmacol.* 1990 Apr.;341(4):308-15.

[12] Butcher, R. W., Baired, C. Effects of prostaglandins on adenosine 3′,5′-monophospate levels in fat and other tissues. *J. Biol. Chem.* 1968; 243: 1713-17.

[13] Bergström, S., et al. The prostaglandins: a family of biologically active lipids. *Pharmacol. Rev.* 1968;(20)1:1-48.

[14] Muller, B., et al. Action of stable prostacycline analogue iloprost on microvascular tone and permeability in the hamster cheek pouch. *Prostgl. Leukotr. Med.* 1987;29:187-98.

[15] Creutzig, A., et al. Muscle tissue oxygen pressure fields and transcutaneous oxygen pressure in healthy men during intra-arterial prostaglandin E$_1$ infusion. *Int. Angiol.* 1984;S3:105

[16] Vaugham, D. E. PGE$_1$ accelerates thrombolysis by tissue plasminogen activator. *Blood* 1989 Apr.;73(5):1213-7.

[17] Loesberg, C., et al. Cell cycle-dependent inhibition of human vascular smooth muscle cell proliferation by prostaglandin E$_1$. *Experimental Cell Research* 1985;160(1):117-25.

[18] Norwegian Pentoxifylline Multicenter Trial Group. Efficacy and clinical tolerance of parenteral pentoxifylline in the treatment of critical lower limb ischemia. A placebo controlled multicenter study. *Int. Angiol.* 1996;15(1):75-80.

[19] Katenschlager, R., et al. Synergism between PGE$_1$-metabolites and nitric oxide on platelet aggregation. *Prostaglandins Leukot. Essent. Fatty Acids* 1992; 45:207-10.

[20] Virgolini, I., et al. Effect of prostaglandin E$_1$ on low density lipoprotein Apo-B,E-receptor binding. *Prostaglandins* 1991;42:81-93.

[21] *Sinzinger, H., Fitscha, P. Influence of prostaglandin E$_1$ on in-vivo accumulation of radio-labeled platelets and LDL in human arteries. VASA-Suppl. 1987;17:5-10.*

[22] Schrör, K., Hohlfeld, T. Mechanisms of anti-ischemic action of prostaglandin E$_1$. *VASA* 2004; 33:119-24.

[23] Gianetti, J., et al. Intravenous Prostaglandin E$_1$ reduces soluble vascular cell adhesion molecule-1 in peripheral arterial obstructive disease. *Am. Heart J.* 2001;142:733-9.

[24] Palumbo, B., et al. Prostaglandin E$_1$-therapy reduces circulating adhesion molecules (ICAM-1, E-selectin, VCAM-1) in peripheral vascular disease. *VASA* 2000;29:179-85.

[25] Sinzinger, H., et al. Pathomechanisms of atherosclerosis beneficially affected by prostaglandin E$_1$ (PGE$_1$) - an update. *Vasa Suppl.* 1989;28:6-13.

[26] Fang, W., et al. Protective effects of prostaglandin E$_1$ on human umbilical vein endothelial cell injury induced by hydrogen peroxide. *Acta Pharmacologica Sinica* 2010; 31:485–92.

[27] Robert, A., et al. Inhibition of gastric secretion by prostaglandins. *Am. J. Dig. Dis.* 1967;12:1073-6.

[28] Watkingson, G., et al. The therapeutic efficacy of Misoprostol in peptic ulcer disease. *Postgrad. Med. J.* 1988;64 (suppl. 1):60-77

[29] Tang, O. S., et al. Misoprostol: Pharmacokinetic profiles, effects on the uterus and side effects. *Int. J. Gynaecol. Obstet.* 2007;99(suppl. 2):S160-7.

[30] Hammerman, C. Patent ductus arteriosus. Clinical relevance of prostaglandins and prostaglandin inhibitors in PDA pathophysiology and treatment. *Clin. Perinatol.* 1995; 22(2):457-79.

[31] Urciuoli, R., et al. Prostaglandin E1 for treatment of erectile dysfunction. *Cochrane Database of Systematic Reviews* 2004, Issue 2. Art. No.: CD 001784.

[32] Fontaine, R., et al. Die chirugische Behandlung der peripheren Durchblutungsstörungen (Surgical treatment of peripheral circulation disorders). In German. *Helvetica Chirurgica Acta* 1954;21:499–533.

[33] Criqui, M. H., et al. The prevalence of peripheral arterial disease in a defined population. *Circulation* 1985;71:510-51.

[34] Hiatt, W. R., et al. Effect of diagnostic criteria on the prevalence of peripheral arterial disease. The San Luis Valley Diabetes Study. *Circulation* 1995;91:1472-9.

[35] Selvin, E., Erlinger, T. P. Prevalence of and risk factors for peripheral arterial disease in the United States: results from the National Health and Nutrition Examination Survey, 1999–2000. *Circulation* 2004;110:738-43.

[36] Hirsch, A. T., et al. ACC/AHA 2005 guidelines for the management of patients with peripheral arterial disease (lower extremity, renal, mesenteric, and abdominal aortic): Executive summary. *J. Am. Coll. Cardiol.* 2006;47:1239–1312.

[37] Dormandy, J., et al. The natural history of claudication: risk of the life and limb. *Semin. Vasc. Surg.* 1999;12:123-37.

[38] Coffman, J. D. Intermittent claudication - be conversative. *N Eng. J. of Med.* 1991; 325: 577-8.

[39] Ernst, E., Fialka, V. A review of the clinical effectiveness of exercise therapy for intermittent claudication. *Archives of Internal Medicine* 1993;153:2357-60. [2090] Leng, G. C., et al. Exercise for intermittent claudication (Cochrane Review). In: *The Cochrane Library*, 2, 2000. Oxford: Update Software. CD000990. [2100] de la Haye, R., et al. An epidemiologic study of the value and limits of physical therapy/exercise therapy in Fontaine stage II arterial occlusive disease. *Vasa Suppl.* 1992; 38:1-40.

[40] Blume, J., et al. Clinical and haemorheological efficacy of i.a. PGE1 infusions in intermittent claudication. *VASA Suppl.* 1987;17:32-5.

[41] Rudofsky, G., et al. Intra-arterial perfusion with prostaglandin E1 in patients with intermittent claudication. *VASA Suppl.* 1987;17:47-51, Rudofsky, G. In: Heidrich, H., Böhme, H., Rogatti, W., editor(s). Prostaglandin E1 - Wirkungen und therapeutische Wirksamkeit. Berlin: Springer - Verlag, 1988:103-11.

[42] Diehm, C., et al. Efficacy of a new prostaglandin E1 regimen in outpatients with severe intermittent claudication: results of a multicenter placebo-controlled double-blind trial. *Journal of Vascular Surgery* 1997; 25:537-44.

[43] Mangiafico, R. A., et al. Impact of a 4-week treatment with prostaglandin E1 on health-related quality of life of patients with intermittent claudication. *Angiology* 2000; 51 (6): 441-9.

[44] Hepp, W., et al. Clinical efficacy of iv Prostaglandin E1 and iv Pentoxifylline in patients with arterial occlusive disease of Fontaine stage IIb: a multicenter, randomized comparative study. *Int. J. Angiol.* 1996;5;32-7.

[45] Scheffler, P., et al. Intensive vascular training in stage IIb of peripheral arterial occlusive disease. The additive effects of intravenous prostaglandin E1 or intravenous pentoxifylline during training. *Circulation* 1994;90:818-22.

[46] Diehm, C., et al. Effects of regular physical training in a supervised class and additional intravenous prostaglandin E1 and naftidrofuryl infusion therapy in patients with intermittent claudication. *Vasa Suppl.* 1989; 28: 20-30.

[47] Belcaro, G., et al. Treatment of severe intermittent claudication with PGE₁. A short-term vs a long-term infusion plan. A 20 week, European randomized trial. Analysis of efficacy and costs. *Angiology* 1998;49: 885-94.

[48] Belch, J. J., et al. Randomized, double-blind, placebo-controlled study evaluating the efficacy and safety of AS-013, a prostaglandin E1 prodrug, in patients with intermittent claudication. *Circulation* 1997; 95: 2298-302.

[49] Lièvre, M., et al. Oral Beraprost Sodium, a prostaglandin I(2) analogue, for intermittent claudication: a double blind, randomized, multicenter controlled trial. *Circulation* 2000; 102:426-31.

[50] Setacci, C. Critical Limb Ischemia. *New developments and perspectives.* Turin: Edizioni Minerva Medica; 2010.

[51] Task II Working Group. Inter-Society Consensus for the Management of Peripheral Arterial Disease (TASC II). *Eur. J. Vasc. Endovasc. Surg.* 2007;33:S1-S75.

[52] Gruss, J. D., et al. Conservative treatment of inoperable arterial occlusions of the lower extremities with intra-arterial prostaglandin E1. *Br. J. Surg.* 1982;69 Suppl.:S11-3.

[53] Trübestein, G., et al. Prostaglandin E1 in chronic arterial disease. A multicenter study. *Vasa Suppl.* 1987;17:39-43.

[54] Balzer, K., et al. Efficacy and tolerability of intra-arterial and intravenous prostaglandin E1 infusions in occlusive arterial disease stage III/IV. *Vasa Suppl.* 1989;28:31-8.

[55] Diehm, C., et al. Clinical effects of intravenously administered prostaglandin E1 in patients with rest pain due to peripheral obliterative arterial disease (POAD)--a preliminary report on a placebo-controlled double-blind study. *Vasa Suppl.* 1987;17:52-6.

[56] Trübestein, G., et al. Intravenous prostaglandin E1 versus pentoxifylline therapy in chronic arterial occlusive disease--a controlled randomised multicenter study. *Vasa Suppl.* 1989;28:44-9.

[57] Stiegler, H., et al. Placebo controlled, double-blind study of the effectiveness of i.v. prostaglandin E1 in diabetic patients with stage IV arterial occlusive disease. *Vasa Suppl.* 1992;35:164-6.

[58] Creutzig, A., et al. Meta-analysis of randomized controlled prostaglandin E1 studies in peripheral arterial occlusive disease stages III and IV. *Vasa.* 2004;33(3):137-44.

[59] Hummers, L. K., Wigley, F. M. Management of Raynaud's phenomenon and digital ischemic lesions in scleroderma. *Rheum. Dis. Clin. North Am.* 2003;29:293–313.

[60] Bartolone, S., et al. Efficacy evaluation of prostaglandin E1 against placebo in patients with progressive systemic sclerosis and significant Raynaud's phenomenon. *Minerva Cardioangiol.* 1999;47(5):137-43.

[61] Marasini, B., Massarotti, M., Bottasso, B., et al. Comparison between iloprost and alprostadil in the treatment of Raynaud's phenomenon. *Scand. J. Rheumatol.* 2004; 33:253–256.

[62] Lamprecht, P., et al. Efficacy of alprostadil and iloprost in digital necrosis due to secondary Raynaud's phenomenon. *Br. J. Rheumatol.* 1998;37(6):703-4.

[63] Mohrland, J. S., et al. A multiclinic, placebo-controlled, double-blind study of prostaglandin E1 in Raynaud's syndrome. *Ann. Rheum. Dis.* 1985 Nov.; 44(11):754-60.

[64] Wigley, F. M., et al. Intravenous iloprost treatment of Raynaud's phenomenon and ischemic ulcers secondary to systemic sclerosis. *J. Rheumatol.* 1992; 19: 1407-14.

[65] Lapinskas, V. A brief history of ergotism: From St. Anthony's fire and St. Vitus dance until today. *Medicinos teorija ir praktika* 2007;13(2)202-6.

[66] Dilme-Muñoz, J. F., et al. Ergotismo: revisión de la bibliografía y presentación de casos (Ergotism: Review of the literature and some case reports). In Spanish. *Angiología* 2003;55(4):311-21.

[67] Arkkila, P. E. Thromboangiitis obliterans (Buerger's disease). *Orphanet J. Rare Dis.* 2006;1:14.

[68] Fissinger, J. N., Schäfer, M. Trial of Iloprost versus aspirintreatment for critical limb ischemia of thromboangiitisobliterans. *The Lancet* 1990; 10:555-7.

[69] Choe, H., et al. Intravenous regional administration of prostaglandin E_1 for the treatment of Buerger's disease. *J. Korean Pain Soc.* 1992;5(1):85-88.

[70] Pacifico, F., et al. PGE_1 therapy for Martorell's ulcer. *International Wound Journal* 2011;8(2)140-4.

[71] Garelli, G., et al. Úlcera de Martorell (Martorell's ulcer). In Spanish. *Flebologia y linfologia: Lecturas vasculares* 2009;4(12)737-42.

[72] Borges, M. V., et al. Synthetic prostaglandin treatment in systemic cholesterol crystals embolism following endovascular aneurysm repair. *J. Vasc. Bras.* 2012;11(1):77-82.

[73] González-Gay, M., et al. Prostaglandinas en el tratamiento de la isquemia aguda secundaria a contusion arterial infrapoplítea (Prostaglandins in the treatment of acute ischaemia secondary to an infrapopliteal artery contusion). In Spanish. *Angiologia* 2010;62:33-5.

[74] Weiss, T., et al. Intraindividual evaluation of the optimal PGE_1 application route in critical limb ischemia. *Int. J. Angiol.* 1994;3(1):191-4.

[75] Balzer, K., et al. Efficacy and tolerability of intra-arterial and intravenous prostaglandin E_1 infusions in occlusive arterial disease stage III/IV. *VASA* 1989;28:31-8.

[76] Heidrich, H., et al. Long-term intravenous infusion of PGE1 in peripheral arterial blood flow disorders: results of an open screening study with patients in Fontaine's stages III and IV. In: Sinzinger, H. and Rogatti, W. *Prostaglandin E in atherosclerosis*. Springer Verlag, Berlin 1986:92-8.

[77] Belcaro, G., et al. PGE1 treatment of severe intermittent claudication (short-term versus long-term, associated with exercise)--efficacy and costs in a 20-week, randomized trial. *Angiology* 2000 Aug.; 51(8 Pt 2):S15-26.

In: Advances in Medicine and Biology. Volume 69
Editor: Leon V. Berhardt

ISBN: 978-1-62808-088-9
© 2013 Nova Science Publishers, Inc.

Chapter III

Expression and Involvement of Cytokines, Chemokines and Adhesion Molecules in Rheumatoid Vasculitis

Tsuyoshi Kasama[1]*, Kumiko Ohtsuka[1], Kuninobu Wakabayashi[1], Takeo Isozaki[1] and Kazuo Kobayashi[2]

[1]Division of Rheumatology, Department of Medicine,
Showa University School of Medicine, Tokyo
[2]Department of Immunology, National Institute of Infectious Diseases, Tokyo, Japan

Abstract

Rheumatoid vasculitis (RV) is an uncommon but severe complication of rheumatoid arthritis (RA) that can cause skin disorders, such as rashes, cutaneous ulcerations, gangrene, neuropathy, eye symptoms, and systemic inflammation. Although the molecular mechanisms underlying RV are unclear, it is well known that a chronic imbalance in the expression of chemokines and proinflammatory cytokines facilitates inflammatory responses in RA patients. Dysregulation of cytokines and other inflammatory molecules, such as adhesion molecules, has also been suggested to occur in patients with RV. Recently, we reported elevated levels of the chemokine CX3CL1 and macrophage migration inhibitory factor in the serum of patients with RV. In this chapter, we discuss the involvement of cytokines and inflammatory molecules in the pathogenesis of RV and evaluate their significance as useful laboratory parameters of active vasculitis disease.

* Reprint requests: Tsuyoshi Kasama, MD, PhD, Division of Rheumatology, Department of Medicine, Showa University School of Medicine, 1-5-8 Hatanodai, Shinagawa-ku, Tokyo 142-8666, Japan. Fax: +81-33784-8742, E-mail address: tkasama@med.showa-u.ac.jp

Keywords: rheumatoid vasculitis, cytokines, chemokines, adhesion molecules

Introduction

Rheumatoid vasculitis (RV) is an uncommon but severe complication of rheumatoid arthritis (RA) that can cause skin disorders, neuropathy, eye symptoms, and systemic inflammation [1, 2].

Although it is well known that chronically imbalanced expression of cytokines and chemokines facilitates the inflammatory responses observed in the pathology of RA patients [3-6], the pathogenesis of RV has not been fully elucidated. The present section discusses the involvement of cytokines and inflammatory molecules in the pathogenesis of RV and evaluates their significance as useful laboratory parameters of active vasculitis disease.

Endothelial Cells and Inflammatory Cells Are Main Players in Vasculitis

Although the causes of most vasculitis syndromes remain unclear, advances in molecular and cellular immunology have defined many of the effector mechanisms that mediate inflammatory vascular damage. Endothelial cells (ECs) play a pivotal role in the pathogenesis of systemic vasculitis, and vascular endothelial dysfunction is common in a variety of immune-mediated inflammatory diseases, such as vasculitis [7-9]. RV is defined histologically as the presence of vasculitis with an inflammatory infiltrate and destruction of the vessel wall [2, 10, 11].

These changes result from circulating immune complexes containing rheumatoid factor (RF) and autoantibodies that form deposits on vessel walls and trigger an inflammatory reaction, which may lead to EC injury and activation [12, 13]. ECs have significant proinflammatory activities and secrete and express various cytokines, chemokines, cell adhesion molecules, and other inflammatory molecules [14].

ECs are involved in cell-cell interactions, especially with invading mononuclear cells, which suggests a pivotal role in the progression of vasculitis and autoimmune diseases such as RA and systemic lupus erythematosus (SLE).

Cytokines

Cytokines play a key role in the pathogenesis of RA, both in systemic inflammatory processes, such as the upregulation of acute-phase protein synthesis, and in the effects of cytokines in the vascular endothelium, which lines the vessels [15-18].

The vascular endothelium is the primary target of circulating mediators and thus controls cell and molecule trafficking from the bloodstream into the underlying tissue. Cross-talk between ECs, leucocytes, and cytokines serves a homeostatic function and acts as a rapid response facility during vascular injury, which is commonly observed in RV and systemic vasculitis.

TNF-α

Tumor necrosis factor (TNF) is considered to be a primary cytokine in chronic, destructive arthritis, such as RA, although there are many other proinflammatory cytokines known to play a role in the pathogenesis of vasculitis syndrome and RA [19, 20]. To date, therapeutic approaches to RA patients have focused on TNF, which is a major inflammatory mediator in RA and a potent inducer of IL-1. Targeted inhibition of TNF-α is an effective therapy in patients with RA [15, 21, 22]. Recently, increasing evidence has indicated that TNF-α, a cytokine that activates the vascular endothelium, also plays a key role in the pathophysiology of vascular involvement in RA. Immunoreactive TNF-α and intercellular adhesion molecule (ICAM)-1 were significantly expressed in ECs and perivascular cellular infiltrate within labial salivary glands from patients with active RV both independently and possibly in combination with RA and Sjögren's syndrome [23]. Interestingly, TNF expression in salivary glands decreased or disappeared following successful treatment. Kuryliszyn-Moskal [24] examined the serum levels of TNF-α, IL-6, soluble CD4 (sCD4), sCD8, and sIL-6 receptor (sIL-6R) in RA patients to evaluate the relationship between extra-articular manifestations (EAMs), such as peripheral neuropathy, skin ulcers, necrotizing glomerulonephritis, fibrosing alveolitis, ischemic colitis, nailfold lesions, pericarditis, pleuritis, (epi-)scleritis, weight loss, fever and multiple rheumatoid nodules, and immunological alterations. The serum levels of TNF-α, sIL-6, sIL-6R, and sCD4 were significantly higher in RA patients compared to healthy subjects. In addition, RA patients exhibiting clinical signs of vasculitis demonstrated significantly higher levels of TNF-α and IL-6 compared to patients without vascular involvement. Furthermore, Turesson et al. also observed higher levels of TNF in patients with systemic vasculitis compared to those without any evidence of systemic involvement [25]. Although anti-TNF therapy effectively decreased the disease activity and synovial inflammation associated with RA, cutaneous vasculitis developed as a complication [26-29]. Recently, Srivastava et al. observed dysregulated expression of cytokines and chemokines in cutaneous lymphocytic vasculitis in patients with Crohn's disease but not RA [30].

In this report, elevated expression levels of RANTES, eotaxin, IL-15, IL-16 and IL-18 were detected with exacerbation of vasculitis after treatment with infliximab, which indicates the polarization of the Th1-skewed inflammatory response. Together, these results demonstrate that TNF-α has an important role in the cytokine network in RV pathogenesis, as well as in RA, and suggest an important role for cellular immune activation in the pathogenesis of microvascular damage.

IL-6

IL-6 plays an important role in the regulation of inflammatory and immune responses and hematopoiesis, including B cell maturation, immunoglobulin production, induction of acute phase proteins in the liver, and T cell maturation and activation [31, 32]. Based on the potential contribution of IL-6 to immune responses, especially B cell maturation and immunoglobulin production, numerous studies have investigated the contribution of IL-6 to the development of autoimmune disorders, such as SLE, which are characterized by the dysregulated production of autoantibodies and polyclonal B cell activation [33]. Cumulative evidence has shown that IL-6 is an important mediator of RA disease [32, 34]. Although IL-6 plays a crucial role in the inflammatory condition and immune-mediated diseases, little information is available on IL-6 expression in vasculitis [35, 36]. Kuryliszyn-Moskal observed increased IL-6 levels in RA patients with vascular involvement [24]. As mentioned previously, the serum levels of IL-6 and its specific soluble receptor sIL-6R, TNF-α, and sCD4 were significantly higher in RA patients compared to healthy subjects. RA patients with clinical signs of systemic vasculitis exhibited significantly higher levels of IL-6 compared to patients without vascular involvement. The statistical analyses of all of the RA patients, with and without vasculitis, demonstrated significant correlations between IL-6 and sCD4 and sCD8, as well as the erythrocyte sedimentation rate (ESR). Although the IL-6 and sIL-6R levels were significantly higher in RA patients than in the healthy controls, no significant differences were observed between the RA groups with and without vasculitis. Furthermore, there was no association between the severity of microvascular damages and the levels of IL-6 and sIL-6R [24]. These results showing the lack of a correlation between IL-6 or sIL-6R and vasculitis complications in RA patients suggest that the IL-6/IL-6R systems might be regulated during the development of vasculitis by different mechanisms or RV disease stages.

Chemokines

Chemokines are known to belong to two major superfamilies that share substantial homology via four conserved cysteine residues [16, 37, 38]. The CXC chemokine family [e.g., CXCL1 (growth related oncogene alpha; GRO-α), CXCL5 (expression of neutrophil activating protein-78; ENA-78), CXCL8 (IL-8), CXCL9 (monokine induced by interferon-gamma; MIG), CXCL10 (interferon-inducible protein 10; IP-10), CXCL11 (interferon-inducible T cell A chemoattractant; I-TAC) and CXCL16 (CXC chemokine ligand 16)] induces chemotaxis mainly in neutrophils and T lymphocytes, whereas the CC chemokine family [e.g., CCL2 (macrophage chemoattractant protein 1; MCP-1), CCL3 (macrophage inflammatory protein 1 alpha; MIP-1α) and CCL5 (regulated on activation normal T cells expressed and secreted; RANTES)] induces chemotaxis in monocytes and subpopulations of T lymphocytes. CX3CL1 (fractalkine) has also been identified. The members of these families demonstrate considerable structural homology and often possess overlapping chemoattractant specificities.

In addition to their roles in chemoattraction, chemokines have been implicated in rheumatic disorders, including RA and SLE [6, 39]. Although multiple studies have documented the localization of various chemokines in pathological conditions, such as systemic vasculitis [40-42], there is no published evidence of the involvement of other chemokines in RV without CX3CL1 and macrophage migration inhibitory factor (MIF), which are described in the next section.

CX3CL1

CX3CL1, also known as fractalkine, is synthesized as a type I transmembrane protein by ECs [43]. The soluble form of CX3CL1 reportedly exerts a chemotactic effect on monocytes, NK cells, and T lymphocytes. CX3CL1 acts via its receptor, CX3CR1, as an adhesion molecule that is able to promote firm adhesion of a subset of leukocytes to ECs under conditions of physiological flow [44, 45]. Thus, CX3CL1 appears to possess immunoregulatory properties, which affects inflammatory and immune cell-EC interactions and inflammatory responses at the inflamed sites. Indeed, numerous studies have implicated CX3CL1 in a variety of inflammatory disorders, including glomerulonephritis, RA, systemic sclerosis, and SLE [46-51]. We have demonstrated significant expression of CX3CL1 in RV [52]. In that report, patients with RA were classified into three groups: the RA group, the EAM-RA group, and the RV group. The serum CX3CL1 levels were significantly higher in the RV group and the EAM-RA group compared to the RA group. Furthermore, in the RV group, there were significant correlations between the CX3CL1 levels and the disease activity scores for vasculitis and significant positive and negative correlations with serum immune complex and serum complement levels. The CX3CL1 levels in the RV patients were significantly correlated with the ICAM-1 levels, which indicate endothelial damage and/or vascular inflammation [53-55]. The accumulation of activated cells and the upregulated expression of inflammatory molecules, including ICAM-1 and CX3CL1, reflect the pathophysiological events leading to vasculitis. In addition, we clearly showed that cellular localization of CX3CL1 protein could be identified in ECs in vasculitic arteries using immunohistochemical analysis. Furthermore, the mRNA expression of CX3CL1 was significantly greater in peripheral blood mononuclear cells from active RV patients than from RA patients and controls. Notably, the serum CX3CL1 levels were significantly diminished following successful treatment and clinical improvement. These results suggest that the level of CX3CL1 in serum influences the magnitude of activation and inflammation of ECs. The higher CX3CL1 levels in RV patients compared to RA or EAM-RA patients might be interpreted as an indicator of undiagnosed vasculitis in RA patients or may support the hypothesis that vasculopathy underlies EAMs in RA. Recently, Bjerkeli et al. showed that the serum levels of CX3CL1 in patients with Wegener's granulomatosis (WG) were significantly increased compared with healthy controls [56]. Along with our results from RV [52], these results suggest that the level of CX3CL1 in serum indicates the magnitude of activation and inflammation of ECs in small vessel vasculitis in WG and especially RV. TNF-α stimulation of ECs significantly and potently induces CX3CL1 [57, 58]. Increasing evidence suggests that by mediating vascular endothelial activation, TNF-α plays a key role in the pathophysiology of systemic vasculitis [1, 59]. Dysregulation of cytokine networks between CX3CL1 and inflammatory cytokines, especially TNF-α, may impact the development of RV.

MIF

Macrophage migration inhibitory factor (MIF) was originally identified as a soluble factor in the culture medium of activated T lymphocytes and inhibited the random migration of macrophages. It is now recognized as a multipotent cytokine in the regulation of immune and inflammatory responses [60] and is known to be a broad-spectrum intracellular and extracellular protein produced by a variety of cell types [61, 62]. The pleiotropic nature of MIF is illustrated by the numerous mechanisms implicated in its effects, including the activation of mitogen-activated protein kinase (MAPK) signaling [63], the upregulation of proinflammatory mediators [61], the counterregulation of endogenous glucocorticoids [64, 65] and the inhibition of apoptosis [66]. Moreover, MIF has been implicated in various inflammatory and immune-mediated diseases, including RA [67, 68], SLE [68, 69], scleroderma [69], ankylosing spondylitis [70], and inflammatory bowel diseases [71]. Recently, we have shown that increased serum MIF levels were also associated with systemic vasculitis, including microscopic polyangiitis [72]; these conditions are strongly associated with anti-neutrophil cytoplastic antibody (ANCA). Notably, significantly elevated levels of serum MIF were observed in patients with microscopic polyangiitis (MPA), which is a small vessel vasculitis, but not in patients with medium vessel vasculitis, such as polyarteritis nodosa, or large vessel vasculitis, such as giant cell arteritis and Takayasu aortitis [72]. The elevated MIF levels in MPA patients correlated positively with indexes of disease activity, including Birmingham vasculitis activity scores, CRP levels and ESR. Furthermore, the MIF levels were significantly diminished in MPA patients exhibiting clinical improvement after treatment. Similarly, the serum MIF levels were elevated in patients with ANCA-related vasculitis [73], Wegener's granulomatous and Kawasaki disease [74]. These findings indicate that MIF expression is not specific to RA but may also function as an important regulator of systemic vasculitis. In patients with MPA, the origin of the elevated serum MIF appears to be ECs and/or inflammatory cells such as monocytes and polymorphonuclear neutrophils [75, 76]. After it is secreted, MIF likely regulates EC proliferation [77]. There was also a positive correlation between the serum MIF levels and MPO-ANCA titers in MPA patients [72]. Although there are no data reporting the capacity of MPO-ANCA to stimulate secretion of any cytokine, including MIF, we would expect it to be related to disease activity and MIF levels because there appears to be positive relationship between MPO-ANCA titers and vasculitis disease activity [78]. As mentioned earlier, MIF upregulates ICAM-1 in ECs [79] and upregulates the expression and secretion of other inflammatory cytokines, including TNF-α and IL-8 [67, 80]. These mechanisms would be expected to enhance the recruitment of leukocytes to sites of inflammation, which involves adhesion molecule-dependent interactions with ECs. Recently, we reported significantly higher serum levels of MIF in patients with RV than in those without RV [81]. We found significant positive correlations in RV patients between the MIF levels and vasculitis disease activity scores and the serum levels of immune complex. We also observed a significant negative correlation between the MIF levels and serum complement levels. Notably, the MIF levels in RV patients also correlated significantly with levels of thrombomodulin, which is associated with endothelial damage and/or vascular inflammation. In conclusion, in the vasculitis patients, the MIF levels were significantly higher in patients in the small vessel vasculitis group than in the other groups. RV is categorized as small-vessel vasculitis. Collectively, these findings suggest that dysregulated actions of MIF, adhesion molecules and cytokines expressed by ECs and/or leukocytes play a crucial role in the development of systemic vasculitis (e.g., MPA and RV).

Adhesion and Related Molecules

Adhesion molecules, such as ICAM-1, vascular cell adhesion molecule-1 (VCAM-1), and other related molecules, are thought to mediate intercellular adhesion. Adhesion is mediated through a variety of receptors with unique physical and kinetic characteristics, regulatory patterns, and tissue and cell localizations that are well suited to their diverse functions [82]. The adhesion molecules ICAM-1, VCAM-1, and E-selectin are regulated by proinflammatory cytokines and play an important role in the binding and activation of leukocytes in vascular inflammation in RA, SLE and systemic vasculitis [8, 83-85].

ICAM-1

ICAM-1, also known as CD54, is a cell surface glycoprotein that contributes to interactions between leukocytes and several other cell types, including ECs, fibroblasts, and keratinocytes [86-88]. Although ICAM-1 is constitutively expressed by monocytes/macrophages, lymphocytes, and ECs, stimulation of cells with cytokines or microbial infection can induce a marked increase in ICAM-1 expression. ICAM-1 is expressed in rheumatoid synovial tissues [89-91], and the administration of ICAM-1 antibodies in animal models of arthritis slows disease progression [92]. Thus, ICAM-1 may play an important role in the development of inflammatory arthritis. In addition, ICAM-1 and endothelial selectin are expressed on activated endothelium to facilitate localization of leukocytes to the site of vascular injury. A circulating, soluble form of ICAM-1 (sICAM-1) was detected in the serum of patients with RA and systemic vasculitis [54, 93, 94], and *in situ* expression of the ICAM-1 protein in patients with RV has been reported [23]. In that report, ICAM-1 protein, TNF-α, and E-selectin were expressed in ECs and perivascular mononuclear cells in areas of microvascular damage in the salivary glands of RV patients [23]. Furthermore, elevated levels of sICAM-1 were observed in RV patients [53, 95, 96]. RA patients with clinical signs of vasculitis showed significantly higher levels of sICAM-1 than those without vasculitis. Although there was no significant correlation between sICAM-1 levels and capillaroscopic findings, 75% of the patients with severe vascular changes in capillaroscopy exceeded the normal sICAM-1 cut-off value [53]. In addition, Voskuyl et al. [95] demonstrated the involvement of ICAM-3 and ICAM-1 in patients with RV. RV patients had significantly elevated levels of sICAM-1 and sICAM-3 but not sE-selectin compared to RA patients without vasculitis [95]. This result suggests that sICAM-1 and sICAM-3 may be useful markers of vascular inflammation in patients with RV and have a crucial role in the development of vasculitis in RA.

VCAM-1

VCAM-1 recognizes alpha 4 beta 1 integrin and is expressed in all leukocytes except neutrophils [82, 97, 98]. The VCAM-1/alpha 4 beta adhesion pathway has a major effect on eosinophil, lymphocyte, and monocyte trafficking [99-102]. This phenomenon suggests the possibility of creating therapeutic targets to treat various inflammatory disorders and autoimmune diseases by blockade or inhibition of the VCAM-1/alpha 4 beta 1 interaction. In addition to ICAM-1, VCAM-1 has been reported to be clinically involved in RA and systemic vasculitis by several investigators. In RA patients, the VCAM-1 protein was detected in inflamed pannus, particularly on the surface of fibroblasts and infiltrating T lymphocytes [102-104]. In contrast to ICAM-1, studies investigating VCAM-1 in RV and RA are contradictory. Salih et al. [105] reported that RA patients with neuropathy had significantly higher serum levels of sVCAM-1 than patients without neuropathy and healthy controls. In addition, immunohistological analysis revealed significantly greater expression levels of VCAM-1 and ICAM-1 in muscle biopsies from RA patients with vasculitis compared to those without vasculitis [106]. However, VCAM-1 was not detected in vasculitis lesions in the salivary glands of RV patients despite significant expression of ICAM-1 in ECs and perivascular cellular infiltrates [23]. Furthermore, the serum sVCAM-1 levels were lower or unchanged in patients with RA and systemic vasculitis [54]. These findings indicate that the role of VCAM-1 is limited in the pathogenesis of RV and RA compared to ICAM-1.

E-Selectin

The selectin family member E-selectin, also known as endothelial-leucocyte adhesion molecule-1, mediates the early phase of neutrophil binding and the binding of eosinophils, basophils, monocytes, and certain subsets of T cells [107]. The E-selectin protein was detected in the endothelium in RA synovium, predominantly in venules and capillaries. Blann et al. [54] observed elevated levels of sE-selectin in patients with RA, systemic vasculitis, and scleroderma. Significant correlations in RA patients were observed between sICAM and sVCAM, and a significant correlation between sE-selectin and sICAM was observed in patients with systemic vasculitis. Similar to other adhesion molecules and TNF-α, E-selectin protein was significantly more highly expressed in ECs and perivascular cellular infiltrate in labial salivary glands of patients with RV compared to patients with inactive stages of RV, RA, or Sjögren's syndrome [23]. In contrast, Voskuyl et al. [95] reported no significant increases of sE-selectin in patients with RV. Because the expression of E-selectin and other molecules in salivary glands were especially high in patients with active RV, the presence of microvascular damage in salivary gland tissues in patients with RV may reflect limited and specific dissemination of the vascular inflammatory process.

CD40 Ligand

CD40 ligand (CD40L, also called as CD154), a member of the TNF family of transmembrane glycoproteins, is expressed on the surface of recently activated CD4-positive T cells [108]. Activated T lymphocytes expressing CD40L can engage CD40 on ECs to induce the expression of proinflammatory cytokines and adhesion molecules and have may important roles in vascular inflammation [109-111]. In RA patients, the expression of CD40L was detected in synovial and peripheral blood T cells [112]. Tamura et al. [113] reported significantly elevated levels of sCD40L in association with higher titers of rheumatoid factors (RF) in RV patients compared to RA patients without vasculitis. In that report, the plasma levels of CD40L in patients with systemic vasculitis were significantly lower than the levels in RV patients. In contrast, Kim et al. described eosinophilic vasculitis with infiltration of CD40L-positive eosinophils with a marked increase of serum TNF-α [114]. Furthermore, enhanced expression of CD40L on CD4-positive T cells and platelets and increased serum levels of sCD40L were observed in patients with Kawasaki disease, an acute febrile vasculitic syndrome in children [115]. Although few observations have been reported, these findings suggest that sCD40L is a marker of pathogenic B cell activation in RA, which often occurs in cases of vasculitis. CD40L and/or CD40 in B cell-T cell interactions or interactions with other cells may have important pathogenic roles in vasculitis.

Fibronectin

Fibronectin (FN) is a large adhesive glycoprotein located in the extracellular matrix of many tissues [116]. It is also present in body fluids such as synovial fluid (SF) and plasma. FN regulates cellular adhesion and spreading, cell motility, cell growth, differentiation and opsonization via heparin-binding domains [117, 118]. Some splicing variants of FN are expressed in the synovial endothelium in RA, and the expression of these variants is upregulated by the proinflammatory cytokine IL-1 [119]. Soluble FN (sFN) increased in experimental vascular injury and in the serum of patients with active vasculitis syndromes [120, 121]. These observations indicate that sFN reflects inflammation and injury in blood endothelium. Interestingly, sFN may be indicative of vascular injury and/or inflammation in RV [122]. When RA patients were compared to age-matched controls, significant increases in the serum levels of sFN were observed in RA patients with RV and in EAM-RA patients [122]. Those findings suggest that increased levels of sFN are more frequently observed in RA patients with EAMs and particularly in patients with RV. The mechanism of the sFN increases in RV patients remains to be defined. The high sFN levels in RV patients compared to RA patients might be interpreted as an indicator of undiagnosed active vasculitis in RA patients or may support the hypothesis that vasculopathy underlies EAMs in RA. Those studies reflect various levels of tissue inflammation and stimulation of vascular ECs that could ultimately lead to an enhanced release of sFN in the circulation. Serum sFN, in combination with other molecules, such as adhesion molecules and cytokines, may be clinically valuable as a serological marker for RV.

Conclusion

Despite recent advances in the understanding of the pathogenetic mechanisms of RA, the pathophysiology of RV and vasculitis has not yet been fully elucidated. Orchestration of several cytokines and cell-cell interactions may be critical for the development of RV (Figure 1). Table 1 summarizes the detectable cytokines, chemokines and cell adhesion molecules in RV and their correlations with other markers. Because subclinical EC damage and vasculitis are occasionally observed in inflammatory rheumatic diseases, such as RA, it is important to clinically evaluate and diagnose the complications of systemic and localized vasculitis.

The results indicate that the assessment of serum concentrations of cytokines and inflammatory molecules will provide useful clinical information and a method to monitor therapeutic interventions. Further elucidation of complex molecular networks will improve the understanding of the immunopathology of systemic vasculitis and especially vasculitis in RA.

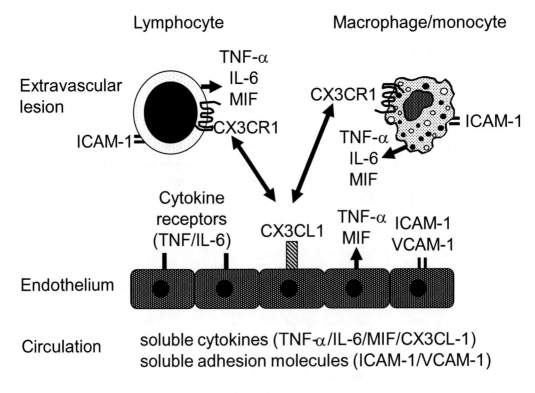

Figure 1. Cytokines/chemokine and cell adhesion molecules involved in RV. Dysregulation and aberrant expression of cytokines and other inflammatory molecules, such as adhesion molecules, in endothelial cells and invading mononuclear cells is pivotal in the progression of RV.

Table 1. Serum levels of soluble cytokines in RA patients with or without vasculitis and correlations with other markers of inflammation

Soluble molecules in serum	Correlated with	References
TNF-α	N.D.	Kuryliszyn-Moskal [24]
	N.D.	Turesson et al. [25]
IL-6	CD4*, CD8*, ESR*	Kuryliszyn-Moskal [24]
CX3CL1	IC, complements	Matsunawa et al. [52]
	Soluble ICAM-1, disease activity	
MIF	IC, complements	Wakabayashi et al. [81]
	Thrombomodulin, disease activity	
ICAM-1	ESR	Kuryliszyn-Moskal [53]
	N.D.	Voskuyl et al. [95],
	Selenium (inverse correlation)	Witkowska et al. [96]
	N.D.	Turesson et al. [25]
VCAM-1	N.D.	Salih et al. [105]
	N.D.	Turesson et al. [25]
CD40 ligand (CD154)	RF	Tamura et al [113]
Fibronectin	disease activity	Voskuyl et al. [122]

*The results of correlations are from all RA patients. N.D., not done; IC, immune complex; ESR, erythrocyte sedimentation rate; TNF-α, tumor necrosis factor-α; MIF, macrophage migration inhibitory factor; ICAM-1, intercellular adhesion molecule-1; VCAM-1, vascular cell adhesion molecule-1; RF, rheumatoid factor.

References

[1]   Genta, MS, Genta RM, Gabay C. Systemic rheumatoid vasculitis: a review. *Semin. Arthritis. Rheum.* 2006; 36: 88-98.

[2]   Turesson, C, Matteson EL. Vasculitis in rheumatoid arthritis. *Curr. Opin. Rheumatol.* 2009; 21: 35-40.

[3]   McInnes, IB, Schett G. Cytokines in the pathogenesis of rheumatoid arthritis. *Nat. Rev. Immunol.* 2007; 7: 429-42.

[4]   Brennan, F, Beech J. Update on cytokines in rheumatoid arthritis. *Curr. Opin. Rheumatol.* 2007; 19: 296-301.

[5]   Kasama, T, Odai T, Wakabayashi K, Yajima N, Miwa Y. Chemokines in systemic lupus erythematosus involving the central nervous system. *Front Biosci.* 2008; 13: 2527-36.

[6]   Szekanecz, Z, Vegvari A, Szabo Z, Koch AE. Chemokines and chemokine receptors in arthritis. *Front Biosci. (Schol. Ed.)* 2010; 2: 153-67.

[7]   Buckley, CD, Rainger GE, Nash GB, Raza K. Endothelial cells, fibroblasts and vasculitis. Rheumatology (Oxford) 2005; 44: 860-3.

[8]   Kaneider, NC, Leger AJ, Kuliopulos A. Therapeutic targeting of molecules involved in leukocyte-endothelial cell interactions. *FEBS Journal* 2006; 273: 4416-24.

[9]   Pate, M, Damarla V, Chi DS, Negi S, Krishnaswamy G. Endothelial cell biology: role in the inflammatory response. *Adv. Clin. Chem.* 2010; 52: 109-30.

[10] Bacons, PA, Kitas GD. The significance of vascular inflammation in rheumatoid arthritis. *Ann. Rheum. Dis.* 1994; 53: 621-3.

[11] Voskuyl, AE, Hazes JM, Zwinderman AH, et al. Diagnostic strategy for the assessment of rheumatoid vasculitis. *Ann. Rheum. Dis.* 2003; 62: 407-13.

[12] Scott, DG, Bacon PA, Allen C, Elson CJ, Wallington T. IgG rheumatoid factor, complement and immune complexes in rheumatoid synovitis and vasculitis: comparative and serial studies during cytotoxic therapy. *Clin. Exp. Immunol.* 1981; 43: 54-63.

[13] Breedveld, FC, Heurkens AH, Lafeber GJ, van Hinsbergh VW, Cats A. Immune complexes in sera from patients with rheumatoid vasculitis induce polymorphonuclear cell-mediated injury to endothelial cells. *Clin. Immunol. Immunopathol.* 1988; 48: 202-13.

[14] Mantovani, A, Dejana E. Cytokines as communication signals between leukocytes and endothelial cells. *Immunol. Today* 1989; 10: 370-5.

[15] Feldmann, M, Brennan FM, Maini RN. Role of cytokines in rheumatoid arthritis. *Annu. Rev. Immunol.* 1996; 14: 397-440.

[16] Kunkel, SL, Lukacs N, Kasama T, Strieter RM. The role of chemokines in inflammatory joint disease. *J. Leukoc. Biol.* 1996; 59: 6-12.

[17] Middleton, J, Americh L, Gayon R, et al. Endothelial cell phenotypes in the rheumatoid synovium: activated, angiogenic, apoptotic and leaky. *Arthritis. Res. Ther.* 2004; 6: 60-72.

[18] Kasama, T, Miwa Y, Isozaki T, Odai T, Adachi M, Kunkel SL. Neutrophil-derived cytokines: potential therapeutic targets in inflammation. *Curr. Drug Targets Inflamm. Allergy* 2005; 4: 273-9.

[19] Cid, MC, Segarra M, Garcia-Martinez A, Hernandez-Rodriguez J. Endothelial cells, antineutrophil cytoplasmic antibodies, and cytokines in the pathogenesis of systemic vasculitis. *Curr. Rheumatol. Rep.* 2004; 6: 184-94.

[20] Muller-Ladner, U, Pap T, Gay RE, Neidhart M, Gay S. Mechanisms of disease: the molecular and cellular basis of joint destruction in rheumatoid arthritis. *Nat. Clin. Pract. Rheumatol.* 2005; 1: 102-10.

[21] Taylor, PC. Anti-cytokines and cytokines in the treatment of rheumatoid arthritis. *Curr. Pharm. Des.* 2003; 9: 1095-106.

[22] Atzeni, F, Doria A, Carrabba M, Turiel M, Sarzi-Puttini P. Potential target of infliximab in autoimmune and inflammatory diseases. *Autoimmun. Rev.* 2007; 6: 529-36.

[23] Flipo, RM, Cardon T, Copin MC, Vandecandelaere M, Duquesnoy B, Janin A. ICAM-1, E-selectin, and TNF alpha expression in labial salivary glands of patients with rheumatoid vasculitis. *Ann. Rheum. Dis.* 1997; 56: 41-4.

[24] Kuryliszyn-Moskal, A. Cytokines and soluble CD4 and CD8 molecules in rheumatoid arthritis: relationship to systematic vasculitis and microvascular capillaroscopic abnormalities. *Clin. Rheumatol.* 1998; 17: 489-95.

[25] Turesson, C, Englund P, Jacobsson LT, et al. Increased endothelial expression of HLA-DQ and interleukin 1alpha in extra-articular rheumatoid arthritis. Results from immunohistochemical studies of skeletal muscle. *Rheumatology (Oxford)* 2001; 40: 1346-54.

[26] McCain, ME, Quinet RJ, Davis WE. Etanercept and infliximab associated with cutaneous vasculitis. *Rheumatology (Oxford)* 2002; 41: 116-7.

[27] Guillevin, L, Mouthon L. Tumor necrosis factor-alpha blockade and the risk of vasculitis. *J. Rheumatol.* 2004; 31: 1885-7.

[28] Scott, DL, Kingsley GH. Tumor necrosis factor inhibitors for rheumatoid arthritis. *N. Engl. J. Med.* 2006; 355: 704-12.

[29] Olsen, NJ, Stein CM. New drugs for rheumatoid arthritis. *N. Engl. J. Med.* 2004; 350: 2167-79.

[30] Srivastava, MD, Alexander F, Tuthill RJ. Immunology of cutaneous vasculitis associated with both etanercept and infliximab. *Scand. J. Immunol.* 2005; 61: 329-36.

[31] Akira, S, Taga T, Kishimoto T. Interleukin-6 in biology and medicine. *Adv. Immunol.* 1993; 54: 1-78.

[32] Nishimoto, N, Kishimoto T. Interleukin 6: from bench to bedside. *Nat. Clin. Pract. Rheumatol.* 2006; 2: 619-26.

[33] Cross, JT, Benton HP. The roles of interleukin-6 and interleukin-10 in B cell hyperactivity in systemic lupus erythematosus. *Inflamm Res.* 1999; 48: 255-61.

[34] Naka, T, Nishimoto N, Kishimoto T. The paradigm of IL-6: from basic science to medicine. *Arthritis. Res.* 2002; 4 Suppl 3: S233-42.

[35] Ohlsson, S, Wieslander J, Segelmark M. Circulating cytokine profile in anti-neutrophilic cytoplasmatic autoantibody-associated vasculitis: prediction of outcome? *Mediators Inflamm.* 2004; 13: 275-83.

[36] Hernandez-Rodriguez, J, Segarra M, Vilardell C, et al. Tissue production of pro-inflammatory cytokines (IL-1beta, TNFalpha and IL-6) correlates with the intensity of the systemic inflammatory response and with corticosteroid requirements in giant-cell arteritis. *Rheumatology (Oxford)* 2004; 43: 294-301.

[37] Baggiolini, M. Chemokines and leukocyte traffic. *Nature* 1998; 392: 565-8.

[38] Moser, B, Wolf M, Walz A, Loetscher P. Chemokines: multiple levels of leukocyte migration control. *Trends. Immunol.* 2004; 25: 75-84.

[39] Bodolay, E, Koch AE, Kim J, Szegedi G, Szekanecz Z. Angiogenesis and chemokines in rheumatoid arthritis and other systemic inflammatory rheumatic diseases. *J. Cell Mol. Med.* 2002; 6: 357-76.

[40] Cid, MC, Vilardell C. Tissue targeting and disease patterns in systemic vasculitis. *Best Pract. Res. Clin. Rheumatol.* 2001; 15: 259-79.

[41] Charo, IF, Taubman MB. Chemokines in the pathogenesis of vascular disease. *Circ. Res.* 2004; 95: 858-66.

[42] Dallos, T, Heiland GR, Strehl J, et al. CCL17/thymus and activation-related chemokine in Churg-Strauss syndrome. *Arthritis. Rheum.* 2010; 62: 3496-503.

[43] Bazan, JF, Bacon KB, Hardiman G, et al. A new class of membrane-bound chemokine with a CX3C motif. *Nature* 1997; 385: 640-4.

[44] Imai, T, Hieshima K, Haskell C, et al. Identification and molecular characterization of fractalkine receptor CX3CR1, which mediates both leukocyte migration and adhesion. *Cell* 1997; 91: 521-30.

[45] Umehara, H, Bloom E, Okazaki T, Domae N, Imai T. Fractalkine and vascular injury. *Trends. Immunol.* 2001; 22: 602-7.

[46] Ruth, JH, Volin MV, Haines GK, 3rd, et al. Fractalkine, a novel chemokine in rheumatoid arthritis and in rat adjuvant-induced arthritis. *Arthritis. Rheum.* 2001; 44: 1568-81.

[47] Blaschke, S, Koziolek M, Schwarz A, et al. Proinflammatory role of fractalkine (CX3CL1) in rheumatoid arthritis. *J. Rheumatol.* 2003; 30: 1918-27.

[48] Hasegawa, M, Sato S, Echigo T, Hamaguchi Y, Yasui M, Takehara K. Up regulated expression of fractalkine/CX3CL1 and CX3CR1 in patients with systemic sclerosis. *Ann. Rheum. Dis.* 2005; 64: 21-8.

[49] Yajima, N, Kasama T, Isozaki T, et al. Elevated levels of soluble fractalkine in active systemic lupus erythematosus: Potential involvement in neuropsychiatric manifestations. *Arthritis. Rheum.* 2005; 52: 1670-5.

[50] Ludwig, A, Weber C. Transmembrane chemokines: versatile 'special agents' in vascular inflammation. *Thromb. Haemost.* 2007; 97: 694-703.

[51] Kasama, T, Sato M, Takahashi R, Odai T, Kobayashi K. The CX3CL1/CX3CR1 axis is a sensitive marker of the response to anti-TNF therapy in patients with rheumatoid arthritis. *J. Clin. Rheumatol. Musculoskel. Med.* 2010; 1: 19-25.

[52] Matsunawa, M, Isozaki T, Odai T, et al. Increased serum levels of soluble fractalkine (CX3CL1) correlate with disease activity in rheumatoid vasculitis. *Arthritis. Rheum.* 2006; 54: 3408-16.

[53] Kuryliszyn-Moskal, A, Bernacka K, Klimiuk PA. Circulating intercellular adhesion molecule 1 in rheumatoid arthritis--relationship to systemic vasculitis and microvascular injury in nailfold capillary microscopy. *Clin. Rheumatol.* 1996; 15: 367-73.

[54] Blann, AD, Herrick A, Jayson MI. Altered levels of soluble adhesion molecules in rheumatoid arthritis, vasculitis and systemic sclerosis. *Br. J. Rheumatol.* 1995; 34: 814-9.

[55] Boehme, MW, Schmitt WH, Youinou P, Stremmel WR, Gross WL. Clinical relevance of elevated serum thrombomodulin and soluble E-selectin in patients with Wegener's granulomatosis and other systemic vasculitides. *Am. J. Med.* 1996; 101: 387-94.

[56] Bjerkeli, V, Damas JK, Fevang B, Holter JC, Aukrust P, Froland SS. Increased expression of fractalkine (CX3CL1) and its receptor, CX3CR1, in Wegener's granulomatosis possible role in vascular inflammation. *Rheumatology (Oxford)* 2007; 46: 1422-7.

[57] Imaizumi, T, Yoshida H, Satoh K. Regulation of CX3CL1/fractalkine expression in endothelial cells. *J. Atheroscler. Thromb.* 2004; 11: 15-21.

[58] Ahn, SY, Cho CH, Park KG, et al. Tumor necrosis factor-alpha induces fractalkine expression preferentially in arterial endothelial cells and mithramycin A suppresses TNF-alpha-induced fractalkine expression. *Am. J. Pathol.* 2004; 164: 1663-72.

[59] Feldmann, M, Pusey CD. Is there a role for TNF-alpha in anti-neutrophil cytoplasmic antibody-associated vasculitis? Lessons from other chronic inflammatory diseases. *J. Am. Soc. Nephrol.* 2006; 17: 1243-52.

[60] Bloom, BR, Shevach E. Requirement for T cells in the production of migration inhibitory factor. *J. Exp. Med.* 1975; 142: 1306-11.

[61] Calandra, T, Roger T. Macrophage migration inhibitory factor: a regulator of innate immunity. *Nat. Rev. Immunol.* 2003; 3: 791-800.

[62] Kasama, T, Ohtsuka K, Sato M, Takahashi R, Wakabayashi K, Kobayashi K. Macrophage migration inhibitory factor: a multifunctional cytokine in rheumatic diseases. *Arthritis* 2011; 2010: 1-10.

[63] Mitchell, RA, Metz CN, Peng T, Bucala R. Sustained mitogen-activated protein kinase (MAPK) and cytoplasmic phospholipase A2 activation by macrophage migration inhibitory factor (MIF). Regulatory role in cell proliferation and glucocorticoid action. *J. Biol. Chem.* 1999; 274: 18100-6.

[64] Calandra, T, Bernhagen J, Metz CN, et al. MIF as a glucocorticoid-induced modulator of cytokine production. *Nature* 1995; 377: 68-71.

[65] Leech, M, Metz C, Bucala R, Morand EF. Regulation of macrophage migration inhibitory factor by endogenous glucocorticoids in rat adjuvant-induced arthritis. *Arthritis. Rheum.* 2000; 43: 827-33.

[66] Mitchell, RA, Liao H, Chesney J, et al. Macrophage migration inhibitory factor (MIF) sustains macrophage proinflammatory function by inhibiting p53: regulatory role in the innate immune response. *Proc. Natl. Acad. Sci. USA* 2002; 99: 345-50.

[67] Leech, M, Metz C, Hall P, et al. Macrophage migration inhibitory factor in rheumatoid arthritis: evidence of proinflammatory function and regulation by glucocorticoids. *Arthritis. Rheum.* 1999; 42: 1601-8.

[68] Santos, LL, Morand EF. Macrophage migration inhibitory factor: a key cytokine in RA, SLE and atherosclerosis. *Clin. Chim. Acta.* 2009; 399: 1-7.

[69] Foote, A, Briganti EM, Kipen Y, Santos L, Leech M, Morand EF. Macrophage migration inhibitory factor in systemic lupus erythematosus. *J. Rheumatol.* 2004; 31: 268-73.

[70] Kozaci, LD, Sari I, Alacacioglu A, Akar S, Akkoc N. Evaluation of inflammation and oxidative stress in ankylosing spondylitis: a role for macrophage migration inhibitory factor. *Mod. Rheumatol.* 2010; 20: 34-9.

[71] de Jong, YP, Abadia-Molina AC, Satoskar AR, et al. Development of chronic colitis is dependent on the cytokine MIF. *Nat. Immunol.* 2001; 2: 1061-6.

[72] Kanemitsu, H, Matsunawa M, Wakabayashi K, et al. Increased serum levels of macrophage migration inhibitory factor (MIF) in patients with microscopic polyangiitis. *Rheumatol. Res. Rev.* 2009; 1.

[73] Becker, H, Maaser C, Mickholz E, Dyong A, Domschke W, Gaubitz M. Relationship between serum levels of macrophage migration inhibitory factor and the activity of antineutrophil cytoplasmic antibody-associated vasculitides. *Clin. Rheumatol.* 2006; 25: 368-72.

[74] Lee, TJ, Chun JK, Yeon SI, Shin JS, Kim DS. Increased serum levels of macrophage migration inhibitory factor in patients with Kawasaki disease. *Scand. J. Rheumatol.* 2007; 36: 222-5.

[75] Calandra, T, Bernhagen J, Mitchell RA, Bucala R. The macrophage is an important and previously unrecognized source of macrophage migration inhibitory factor. *J. Exp. Med.* 1994; 179: 1895-902.

[76] Riedemann, NC, Guo RF, Gao H, et al. Regulatory role of C5a on macrophage migration inhibitory factor release from neutrophils. *J. Immunol.* 2004; 173: 1355-9.

[77] Yang, Y, Degranpre P, Kharfi A, Akoum A. Identification of macrophage migration inhibitory factor as a potent endothelial cell growth-promoting agent released by ectopic human endometrial cells. *J. Clin. Endocrinol. Metab.* 2000; 85: 4721-7.

[78] Sinico, RA, Radice A, Corace C, L DIT, Sabadini E. Value of a new automated fluorescence immunoassay (EliA) for PR3 and MPO-ANCA in monitoring disease activity in ANCA-associated systemic vasculitis. *Ann. N. Y. Acad. Sci.* 2005; 1050: 185-92.

[79] Lin, SG, Yu XY, Chen YX, et al. De novo expression of macrophage migration inhibitory factor in atherogenesis in rabbits. *Circ. Res.* 2000; 87: 1202-8.

[80] Onodera, S, Nishihira J, Koyama Y, et al. Macrophage migration inhibitory factor up-regulates the expression of interleukin-8 messenger RNA in synovial fibroblasts of rheumatoid arthritis patients: common transcriptional regulatory mechanism between interleukin-8 and interleukin-1beta. *Arthritis. Rheum.* 2004; 50: 1437-47.

[81] Wakabayashi, K, Otsuka K, Sato M, et al. Elevated serum levels of macrophage migration inhibitory factor and their significant correlation with rheumatoid vasculitis disease activity. *Mod. Rheumatol.* 2011; (in press).

[82] Gearing, AJ, Hemingway I, Pigott R, Hughes J, Rees AJ, Cashman SJ. Soluble forms of vascular adhesion molecules, E-selectin, ICAM-1, and VCAM-1: pathological significance. *Ann. N. Y. Acad. Sci.* 1992; 667: 324-31.

[83] Sfikakis, PP, Tsokos GC. Clinical use of the measurement of soluble cell adhesion molecules in patients with autoimmune rheumatic diseases. *Clin. Diagn. Lab. Immunol.* 1997; 4: 241-6.

[84] Mousa, SA. Cell adhesion molecules: potential therapeutic and diagnostic implications. *Mol. Biotechnol.* 2008; 38: 33-40.

[85] Langer, HF, Chavakis T. Leukocyte-endothelial interactions in inflammation. *J. Cell Mol. Med.* 2009; 13: 1211-20.

[86] Springer, TA. Adhesion receptors of the immune system. *Nature* 1990; 346: 425-34.

[87] Mackay, CR, Imhof BA. Cell adhesion in the immune system. *Immunol. Today* 1993; 14: 99-102.

[88] Lawson, C, Wolf S. ICAM-1 signaling in endothelial cells. *Pharmacol. Rep.* 2009; 61: 22-32.

[89] Hale, LP, Martin ME, McCollum DE, et al. Immunohistologic analysis of the distribution of cell adhesion molecules within the inflammatory synovial microenvironment. *Arthritis. Rheum.* 1989; 32: 22-30.

[90] Ziff, M. Role of the endothelium in chronic inflammatory synovitis. *Arthritis. Rheum.* 1991; 34: 1345-52.

[91] Johnson, BA, Haines GK, Harlow LA, Koch AE. Adhesion molecule expression in human synovial tissue. *Arthritis. Rheum.* 1993; 36: 137-46.

[92] Kakimoto, K, Nakamura T, Ishii K, et al. The effect of anti-adhesion molecule antibody on the development of collagen-induced arthritis. *Cell Immunol.* 1992; 142: 326-37.

[93] Johnson, PA, Alexander HD, McMillan SA, Maxwell AP. Up-regulation of the endothelial cell adhesion molecule intercellular adhesion molecule-1 (ICAM-1) by autoantibodies in autoimmune vasculitis. *Clin. Exp. Immunol.* 1997; 108: 234-42.

[94] Ara, J, Mirapeix E, Arrizabalaga P, et al. Circulating soluble adhesion molecules in ANCA-associated vasculitis. *Nephrol. Dial. Transplant.* 2001; 16: 276-85.

[95] Voskuyl, AE, Martin S, Melchers L, Zwinderman AH, Weichselbraun I, Breedveld FC. Levels of circulating intercellular adhesion molecule-1 and -3 but not circulating endothelial leucocyte adhesion molecule are increased in patients with rheumatoid vasculitis. *Br. J. Rheumatol.* 1995; 34: 311-5.

[96] Witkowska, AM, Kuryliszyn-Moskal A, Borawska MH, Hukalowicz K, Markiewicz R. A study on soluble intercellular adhesion molecule-1 and selenium in patients with rheumatoid arthritis complicated by vasculitis. *Clin. Rheumatol.* 2003; 22: 414-9.

[97] Zimmerman, GA, Mcintyre TM, Prescott SM. Perspectives series: Cell adhesion in vascular biology. *J. Clin. Invest.* 1996; 98: 1699-702.

[98] Cook-Mills, JM, Marchese ME, Abdala-Valencia H. Vascular cell adhesion molecule-1 expression and signaling during disease: regulation by reactive oxygen species and antioxidants. *Antioxid. Redox. Signal* 2011; 15: 1607-38.

[99] van Dinther-Janssen, AC, Horst E, Koopman G, et al. The VLA-4/VCAM-1 pathway is involved in lymphocyte adhesion to endothelium in rheumatoid synovium. *J. Immunol.* 1991; 147: 4207-10.

[100] Dean, DC, Iademarco MF, Rosen GD, Sheppard AM. The integrin alpha 4 beta 1 and its counter receptor VCAM-1 in development and immune function. *Am. Rev. Respir. Dis.* 1993; 148: S43-6.

[101] Foster, CA. VCAM-1/alpha 4-integrin adhesion pathway: therapeutic target for allergic inflammatory disorders. *J. Allergy Clin. Immunol.* 1996; 98: S270-7.

[102] Matsuyama, T, Kitani A. The role of VCAM-1 molecule in the pathogenesis of rheumatoid synovitis. *Hum. Cell* 1996; 9: 187-92.

[103] Koch, AE, Burrows JC, Haines GK, Carlos TM, Harlan JM, Leibovich SJ. Immunolocalization of endothelial and leukocyte adhesion molecules in human rheumatoid and osteoarthritic synovial tissues. *Lab. Invest.* 1991; 64: 313-20.

[104] Postigo, AA, Garcia-Vicuna R, Diaz-Gonzalez F, Arroyo AG. Increased binding of synovial T lymphocytes from rheumatoid arthritis to endothelial-leukocyte adhesion molecule-1 (ELAM-1) and vascular cell adhesion molecule-1 (VCAM-1). *J. Clin. Invest.* 1992; 89: 1445-52.

[105] Salih, AM, Nixon NB, Dawes PT, Mattey DL. Soluble adhesion molecules and anti-endothelial cell antibodies in patients with rheumatoid arthritis complicated by peripheral neuropathy. *J. Rheumatol.* 1999; 26: 551-5.

[106] Verschueren, PC, Voskuyl AE, Smeets TJ, Zwinderman KH, Breedveld FC, Tak PP. Increased cellularity and expression of adhesion molecules in muscle biopsy specimens from patients with rheumatoid arthritis with clinical suspicion of vasculitis, but negative routine histology. *Ann. Rheum. Dis.* 2000; 59: 598-606.

[107] Vannini, N, Pfeffer U, Lorusso G, Noonan DM, Albini A. Endothelial cell aging and apoptosis in prevention and disease: E-selectin expression and modulation as a model. *Curr. Pharm. Des.* 2008; 14: 221-5.

[108] Elgueta, R, Benson MJ, de Vries VC, Wasiuk A, Guo Y, Noelle RJ. Molecular mechanism and function of CD40/CD40L engagement in the immune system. *Immunol. Rev.* 2009; 229: 152-72.

[109] Miller, DL, Yaron R, Yellin MJ. CD40L-CD40 interactions regulate endothelial cell surface tissue factor and thrombomodulin expression. *J. Leukoc. Biol.* 1998; 63: 373-9.

[110] Thienel, U, Loike J, Yellin MJ. CD154 (CD40L) induces human endothelial cell chemokine production and migration of leukocyte subsets. *Cell Immunol.* 1999; 198: 87-95.

[111] Hassan, GS, Merhi Y, Mourad WM. CD154 and its receptors in inflammatory vascular pathologies. *Trends. Immunol.* 2009; 30: 165-72.

[112] MacDonald, KPA, Nishioka Y, Lipsky PE, Thomas R. Functional CD40 ligand is expressed by T cells in rheumatoid arthritis. *J. Clin. Invest.* 1997; 100: 2404-14.

[113] Tamura, N, Kobayashi S, Kato K, et al. Soluble CD154 in rheumatoid arthritis: Elevated plasma levels in cases with vasculitis. *J. Rheumatol.* 2001; 28: 2583-90.

[114] Kim, SH, Kim TB, Yun YS, et al. Hypereosinophilia presenting as eosinophilic vasculitis and multiple peripheral artery occlusions without organ involvement. *J. Korean. Med. Sci.* 2005; 20: 677-9.

[115] Wang, CL, Wu YT, Liu CA, et al. Expression of CD40 ligand on CD4+ T-cells and platelets correlated to the coronary artery lesion and disease progress in Kawasaki disease. *Pediatrics* 2003; 111: E140-7.

[116] Mao, Y, Schwarzbauer JE. Fibronectin fibrillogenesis, a cell-mediated matrix assembly process. *Matrix Biol.* 2005; 24: 389-99.

[117] Ruoslahti, E. Fibronectin and its receptors. *Annu. Rev. Biochem.* 1988; 57: 375-413.

[118] Schwarzbauer, JE. Alternative splicing of fibronectin: three variants, three functions. *Bioessays.* 1991; 13: 527-33.

[119] Boyle, DL, Shi Y, Gay S, Firestein GS. Regulation of CS1 fibronectin expression and function by IL-1 in endothelial cells. *Cell Immunol.* 2000; 200: 1-7.

[120] Peters, JH, Ginsberg MH, Bohl BP, Sklar LA, Cochrane CG. Intravascular release of intact cellular fibronectin during oxidant-induced injury of the in vitro perfused rabbit lung. *J. Clin. Invest.* 1986; 78: 1596-603.

[121] Peters, JH, Maunder RJ, Woolf AD, Cochrane CG, Ginsberg MH. Elevated plasma levels of ED1+ ("cellular") fibronectin in patients with vascular injury. *J. Lab. Clin. Med.* 1989; 113: 586-97.

[122] Voskuyl, AE, Emeis JJ, Hazes JMW, van Hogezand RA, Biemond I, Breedveld FC. Levels of circulating cellular fibronectin are increased in patients with rheumatoid vasculitis. *Clin. Exp. Rheumatol.* 1998; 16: 429-34.

In: Advances in Medicine and Biology. Volume 69
Editor: Leon V. Berhardt
ISBN: 978-1-62808-088-9
© 2013 Nova Science Publishers, Inc.

Chapter IV

Understanding the Soybean Rust Interaction with Soybeans Using Biotechnology

Arianne Tremblay[1], and Benjamin Matthews[2]*

[1]University of Maryland Baltimore County, Department of Biological Sciences,
Hilltop Circle, Baltimore, US
[2]United States Department of Agriculture, Agricultural Research Service,
Soybean Genomics and Improvement Laboratory,
Baltimore Avenue, Bldg. Beltsville, US

Abstract

United States, Brazil and Argentina are the three biggest producers of soybean in the world withat a combined 180 million metric tons each year. Soybean growing in these countries is susceptible to soybean rust caused by *Phakopsora pachyrhizi* Sydow. With new and emerging biotechnological techniques we may develop new strategies for broadening resistance of soybean to soybean rust. Using these new techniques, scientists can identify and study genes expressed during a plant-pathogen interaction from the perspective of both plant and pathogen to better understand the infection process. The recent development of techniques, such as microarray analysis, high-throughput DNA sequencing and laser capture microdissection, has dramatically improved our ability to identify new genes and to examine gene expression in small samples. Microarrays can be used to study changes in expression of thousands of genes per experiment in infected leaves. The complete soybean genome sequence now available provides a template for analyzing gene expression results from deep sequencing of transcripts during the infection process. Deep sequencing provides unprecedented amounts of data for analysis of the genome and gene expression. Laser capture microdissection allows the isolation of

---

* E-mail: arianne@umbc.edu

specific cells from infected leaf cross-sections that can be analyzed for plant and pathogen gene expression using diverse DNA sequencing approaches. There is still a great lack of knowledge of the function of soybean and fungal genes and their spatial and temporal expression. However, these new techniques will provide new information about pathogen development in its host and the host's response to the pathogen. Some of these plant and fungal genes may be useful to broadening soybean resistance to soybean rust.

Keywords: expressed sequence tags, laser capture microdissection, microarray, pyrosequencing

Abbreviations

dai, days after inoculation;
EST, expressed sequence tags;
hai, hours after inoculation;
LCM, laser capture microdissection;
RT-PCR, reverse transcription real time-polymerase chain reaction;
SBS, sequencing-by-synthesis;
SR, soybean rust;
VIGS, virus induced gene silencing.

Introduction

Phakopsora pachyrhizi Sydow is the causative agent of soybean rust (SR) and is the most devastating disease of soybean in some countries throughout the world. Losses in soybean yield due to SR ranging from 10 to 80% have been reported (Garcia et al. 2008). In a survey, 60% of fields planted with soybean in Brazil during the 2001-2002 growing season had SR present. Fungicide applications are the only efficient method to decrease spreading of the disease, and farmers gained about 60% soybean yield advantage using fungicides during a severe outbreak of SR (Yorinori et al. 2005). In 2004, SR arrived in the continental United States, and its full effect on soybean production in this country is still unknown. Currently 3% of the soybean crop in the U.S. is sprayed with fungicide to deter SR outbreaks. To combat the disease, SR scientists have screened over 1,600 soybean accessions for resistance or tolerance to the rust (Miles et al. 2006, 2008). However, there are many isolates of SR, and genes conferring resistance to all isolates have not been identified. Therefore, it would be useful to develop broad durable resistance to SR using other approaches.

The approach we have taken involves the identification of soybean and SR genes expressed in the soybean leaf inoculated with SR during different stages of the infection process to increase our understanding of the interaction of the plant with the rust at the molecular level. From this we hope to identify genes and proteins that may be useful in broadening resistance through genetic engineering. We have been analyzing changes in gene expression in whole infected leaf samples using microarray and new deep sequencing approaches. Furthermore, we used laser capture microdissection (LCM) to isolate SR infection structures and infected soybean cells at different stages of infection, so that we have only those specific cells for study, while the broad background of uninfected cells are excluded. Genes expressed in these collected cells are identified and their expression is monitored through microarrays and gene sequencing either from Sanger sequencing or using the Illumina Genome Analyzer.

Soybean Gene Expression during an Interaction with Soybean Rust

Microarray Analysis on Whole Infected Leaf

In soybean, five independent loci have been identified that confer resistance to SR, *Rpp1-Rpp65*. Choi et al. (2008) examined gene expression in soybean PI200492 containing *Rpp1*, infected with two specific isolates of SR in independent experiments. One isolate resulted in a susceptible or compatible reaction; the other resulted in a resistant or incompatible reaction. Suppressive subtraction cDNA libraries were made from RNA extracted from this material and 1,728 clones were one-pass sequenced. These expressed sequence tags (ESTs) were compared with sequences in GenBank to identify genes of similar sequence with known function.

The inserts of approximately 7,800 cDNAs, including these cDNAs from the suppressive subtraction libraries along with those of numerous other cDNAs, were printed in triplicate as microarrays to examine gene expression in a compatible and incompatible reaction of SR at 6, 12, 24, 48 hours after inoculation (hai) on soybean. Microarrays also were used to examine gene expression in soybean leaves 72 hai by Panthee et al. (2006 and 2009). Similarly, van de Mortel et al. (2007) used Affymetrix microarrays containing representations of 37,500 soybean genes to study gene expression in soybean leaves susceptible and resistant to SR at numerous time points from 6 hai to 168 hai. Similar data was obtained using both systems. Choi et al. (2008) and van de Mortel et al. (2007) demonstrated that numerous genes in secondary metabolism exhibited differential gene expression. Genes, such as phenylalanine ammonia lyase, cinnamoyl-coA-reductase, and chalcone synthase, were differentially expressed.

In fact, van de Mortel et al. (2007) specifically compared expression profiles of ten genes related to flavonoid biosynthesis to demonstrate their differential expression profiles and suggested that there is a distinct biphasic change in transcript levels during the 168 hours examined.

Furthermore, van de Mortel et al. (2007) identified 127 transcription factor probe sets with altered expression profiles during the course of SR infection. These included transcription factors with WRKY and MYB domains. More recently, Soria-Guerra et al. (2009) identified *Glycine tomentella* genes expressed in resistant and susceptible genotypes over a time-course of infection with SR using a long-oligo soybean microarray. Basically, they identified many genes directly involved in plant defense as highly expressed in a resistant genotype compare to a susceptible genotype.

Laser Capture Microdissection to Increase Spatial Resolution

The above experiments were conducted using whole leaves infected with SR. However, analyzing gene expression in cells at the specific site of infection would eliminate background gene expression occurring in non-infected cells. Thus, many techniques such as fluorescent-activated cell sorting (Herzenberg et al. 2002) and magnetic bead-based cell separation (Yang et al. 2008) were developed to isolate specific cells from a specimen. These techniques have requirements not necessarily easily met using plant cells. Foremost, preparation of single cell suspensions may result in alteration or modification of cellular constituents (Curran and Murray 2005). About fifteenten years ago, at the National Institute of Health, Emmert-Buck and his colleagues developed a new technique named LCM to isolate cells and facilitate the analysis of solid tumors (Emmert-Buck et al. 1996; Simone et al. 1998). LCM is a method for isolating cells of interest from microscopic regions of tissue that has been sectioned. LCM can help to eliminate cross-contamination of desired material from other cells, due to its precision of cutting and harvesting of selected cells. The morphology of the cells can be preserved using proper techniques. LCM is rapid and not technically difficult to accomplish with the proper equipment. Tissue samples can be frozen or embedded in paraffin, or plastic. Tissue samples are sectioned into thin layers and mounted on a special glass slide manufactured for LCM use. These slides are overlaid with a special thermoplastic transfer film. The slide is viewed using a microscope with a laser and computer attachment. The computer directs the mobile slide stage and laser beam. The computer is also used to draw the line where the laser beam is to cut the specimen. The laser beam cuts the sample and the thermoplastic transfer film, thus the sample and underlying film are released from the slide and collected in a cap for further analysis. The unselected cells are left behind. The sample can be used for analyses of DNA, RNA, or protein (Liszewsky 2007).

Laser Capture Microdissection Applications

LCM was first used extensively in medical studies and with animal models. It applications on mammalian cells is well established (Peterson et al. 1998; Wong et al. 2000; Burgoon et al. 2005). LCM also has been used to isolate plant cells. Asano et al. (2002) successfully isolated rice phloem cells and constructed a cDNA library from the RNA extracted from those cells. Kerk et al. (2003) isolated different types of cells from different plant varieties, including maize bundle sheath and mesophyll cells, radish cotyledon cells, *Arabidopsis* leaf mesophyll, palisade, and guard cells. They successfully extracted RNA and obtained consistent RT-PCR results from each group of cells collected. Maize epidermal cells and vascular tissues were collected using LCM and the RNA extracted from these cells was used to study gene expression patterns through microarray analysis (Nakazono et al. 2003). A number of research teams have also used LCM to study gene expression in both organisms during a plant interaction with a pathogen. Over the time-course of a plant-pathogen interaction, many biological events occur in each organism. By analyzing whole plant organs infected with a pathogen, no distinction can be made concerning specifically where these events occur or which cell type is involved. Uninfected tissue can obscure events occurring in infected tissue. Using LCM, specific host and pathogen cells can be isolated during a biotrophic relationship so both sides of the relationship can be analyzed. Cells not involved in the interaction can be eliminated. These studies would allow a better understanding of pathogen development and the interaction of pathogens with their hosts. This knowledge may allow scientists to devise new strategies at the molecular level to control pathogens. LCM has been used routinely to collect soybean cells for gene expression analysis. In soybean-nematode interactions, a lot is known about the cytological aspects of formation of the syncytium, or cells upon which the nematode feeds. But molecular analysis of syncytial cells in resistant and susceptibile plants in has been impeded, because it has been difficult to physically isolate syncytial cells from nearby cells. However, our laboratory has used LCM successfully to collect samples enriched in syncytial cells. The syncytial cells were collected from *Glycine max* cultivar Kent 3 and 8 days after inoculation (dai) with soybean cyst nematode, *Heterodera glycines*.

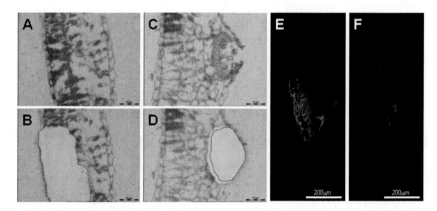

Figure 1. LCM on a longitudinal section of soybean cv. 'Williams 82' leaf inoculated with SR isolate MS06-1. (A) Leaf section with brown coloration into the palisade layer cells 10 dai visualized at 40X magnification (B) Same section visualized after microdissection (C) Uredinium on the lower leaf surface 10 dai visualized at 40X magnification (D) Same section visualized after microdissection (E) Leaf section visualized under a fluorescent filter 24 hai at 10X magnification (F) Same section visualized after microdissection.

WWe determined which genes were expressed in these cells in the resistant and susceptible reactions using expressed sequence tag (EST) sequencing and microarray analysis (Klink et al. 2005, 2007, 2009, 2010a, 2010b, 2011).

In plant-fungus interactions, Hacquard et al. (2010) have been interested to studiedy the uredinial stage of *Melampsora larici-populina* on poplar infected leaves and were ablebe able to separate two contrasted fungal tissues: a biotropic area in the plant mesophyll and a sporulation area below the abaxial epidermis.

Using LCM and microarray technologies, they have been able to pinpoint that there is a massive induction of genes encoding small secreted proteins (SSP) and genes encoding proteins involved in SSP release in the biotrophic area mostly responsible of host defense suppression. In counterpart, in the sporulation area there is a strong induction of genes encoding proteins involved in cell cycle and transport mechanisms in order to translocate metabolites from haustoria to urediniospores needed for cell division and ultimately spore production.

Microarray Analysis on Laser Capture Microdissected SR Infected Soybean Samples

Recently, our laboratory has isolated palisade layer cells from soybean leaveplants. The cells showeding a particular brown coloration at 10 dai with SR using LCM (Figure 1A, 1B). RNA extracted from those cells has been submitted to two-cycle amplification before being used on a Ssoybean Affymetrix chip to identifyied differentially expressed genes in the plant (Tremblay et al. 2010). Most of the genes at this specific time-point are down-regulated. We found that genes involved in the energy production are the most affected.

Transcripts of genes encoding different photosystem subunits as well as glyceraldehyde-3-phosphate dehydrogenase, fructose-bisphosphate aldolase and ribulose bisphosphate carboxylase were decreased in number, as were transcriptgenes encoding several chlorophyll binding proteins. In addition to genes involved in energy production, genes involved in nitrogen metabolism were decreased in expression.

As expected, genes categorized as disease and defense-related weare the most up-regulated. In this category genes encoding for pathogenesis-related protein 10 (PR-10) and disease resistance-responsive protein-related were highly expressed.

Soybean Rust Gene Expression during an Interaction with Soybean Plant

Soybean Rust Gene Expression Analysis Using Sanger DNA Sequencing

LCM has also been used to isolate infection structures from thea biotrophic plant-pathogen interaction ofas soybean and-soybean rust. The isolation of infection structures from a biotrophic fungus is usually associated with a laborious procedure as seen for the isolation of haustoria (Tiburzi et al. 1992; Hahn and Mendgen 1997).

Up to now, the only published studies on SR structures have been on ungerminated and germinated urediniospores. Posada-Buitrago and Frederick (2005) sequenced 908 clones from germinating SR urediniospores and identified 189 sequences with similarity to known sequences using Sanger sequencing. Using LCM we isolated SR uredinia at 10 dai to identify genes associated with uredinium development and urediniospores production (Figure 1.C, 1.D; Tremblay et al. 2008). RNA was extracted from those cells for cDNA library construction and sequencing also using Sanger. We identified several genes that may be associated with the infection process. Through EST sequencing of 925 cDNA clones we determined the identity of a number of genes expressed during the development of the uredinium. Transcripts encoding a nucleosome assembly protein appeared to be the highest expressed among identified genes.

A serine/threonine protein phosphatase and ribosomal protein S17 were also highly expressed. Many other transcripts were expressed; however, the function of most of these transcripts is unknown. This is a serious drawback to defining and understanding the interaction of SR with soybean at the molecular level.

Soybean and Soybean Rust Gene Expression Analysis Using Deep Sequencing Technology

Although sequencing of cDNA libraries using Sanger technology (Sanger et al. 1977) is a reliable method to identify genes expressed in biotrophic fungi, this approach sometimes provides only a very modest number of sequences, especially from material collected using LCM. This limitation is dependent upon the amplification and cloning technology used, bacteria transformation, plasmid purification, and other steps to prepare the sample for sequencing. Also, costs associated with this new technology are fairly high. On the other hand, microarrays can be useful to analyze the expression of soybean genes in leaves during SR infection.

Also, costs associated with this technology are fairly high. On the other hand, microarrays can be useful to analyze the expression of soybean genes in leaves during SR infection.

However, this technology is dependent upon the availability of gene sequences, and it does not allow for gene discovery. Since no commercial microarrays are available for SR, this technology cannot be used to analyze the transcriptome of the fungus without intensive effort. Deep sequencing technologies can bypass some of these problems. Next-generation of sequencing (NGS) can produce millions of DNA sequences from one sample. The sample can contain multiple organisms, and they can be sequenced simultaneously at a fairly low cost to produce data for all organisms in the sample. Differential gene expression analysis can be obtained, and new genes can be identified.

Deep Sequencing Technologies

One of these deep sequencing techniques appeared in 2004. 454 Life Science developed a sequencer based on a sequencing-by-synthesis (SBS) method named pyrosequencing (Margulies et al. 2005). SBS consists of taking a single strand of the DNA to be sequenced and synthesizing its complementary strand enzymatically, one base pair at a time. Then the base that was actually added at each step is identified.

The principle of pyrosequencing lies in the interaction of DNA polymerase with another chemiluminescent enzyme which relies on detection of pyrophosphate release upon nucleotide incorporation rather than chain termination with dideoxynucleotides (Ronaghi 2001). With the 454 sequencer, the template DNA is immobilized on the surface of an agarose bead. Each of the hundreds of thousands beads have a single unique DNA fragment hybridized to it.

Light is produced from the cleavage of oxyluciferine by luciferase only when the nucleotide solution complements the first unpaired base of the template. Depending on the chemiluminescent signal produced, the sequence of the template is determined.

In 2006, Illumina developed a sequencer based on the same SBS concept with the difference that the template DNA is immobilized on the surface of a glass flow cell, and solutions of the differentially labeled fluorescent nucelotides A, C, G, and T, are added and removed sequentially after the reaction (Bennet 2004; Bennet et al. 2005).

These methods greatly reduce the reaction volume while dramatically expanding the number of sequencing reactions. The current 454 instrument produces an average read length of 400 base pair (bp) per bead with a combined throughput of 400 Mb of sequence data per 10-hours run. A typical run on an Illumina sequencer produces 640 million DNA sequence reads of 36 to 150 bp.

By contrast, a single ABI 3730 programmed to sequence 24 96-well plates per day produces only 440 kb of sequence data in 7 hours, with an average read-length of 650 bp per sample. The short read-lengths generated by the Illumina sequencer have raised significant challenges during assembly of DNA contigs due to the vast amount of data generated and the complexity of assembling and annotating this data. All of these companies are working hard to improve read-length. Roche expects to extend read-length to 1,000 bp soon on their 454 instrument.

mRNA Seq Procedure

cDNA as well as genomic DNA can be sequenced by these new technologies. cDNA sequencing is named mRNA-seq. The workflow to produce NGS-ready libraries is straightforward. cDNA is synthesized by standard methods, then DNA fragments are prepared for sequencing by ligating specific adaptor oligos to both ends of each DNA fragment. Importantly, relatively little input DNA is needed to sequence millions of base pairs.

Compared to gene expression studiesy using microarrays, which are limited to sequences present on the arrays, this new sequencing technology is unlimited in its ability to detect genes expressed, and it measures the absolute abundance of transcripts.

Moreover, because a large number of reads is obtained, it is sensitive enough to detect transcription of genes at a low level, which can be missed by EST sequencing analysis (Denoeud et al. 2008). Since they rely on sequence-specific probe hybridization, microarrays also suffer from background and cross-hybridization problems. With deep sequencing technologies, you can obtain DNA sequence representing all transcripts in the sample.

Deep Sequencing Applications

Our laboratory used the Illumina platform to analyze differential gene expression atin diverse infection stages of soybean leaves by SR. We isolated RNA from leaf sections of soybean cultivar Williams 82 containing a mixture of epidermal, palisade and mesophyll soybean cells surrounding a fluorescent signal related to the expression of a SR-secreted protein. Samples were collected at 7, 24 and 48 hai (Figure 1E, 1F) using LCM. mRNAs from these samples were isolated, converted to cDNA, and sequenced using to obtain a view of the whole transcriptome using the Illumina RNA-Seq platform. The data were analyzed to understand gene expression during SR infection of soybean leaves. The lack of genome information for filamentous fungi and SR makes contig assembly and analysis tasks more complicated for SR sequences than other organisms with a sequenced genome, but not impossible. Thousands of contigs were assembled for each time-point, but they were all relatively short with the longest one being 173 bp. Due to their fairly short length, sequence alignment and establishing function, through comparison of the encoded predicted protein with proteins of known function, were difficult to establish and gave high E-values. Table 1.

depicts some of the longest contigs encoding a proteins with similarity to proteins from different protein databases or that encode signal peptides. A gene encoding methylenetetrahydrofolate reductase involved in methionine biosynthesis was expressed at 7 hai. Methionine is one amino acid which is synthesized by the fungus. At 24 hai, the fungus enters its host and begins to multiply, so genes encoding proteins involved in biogenesis of cell walls also were expressed, such as beta-1,3-glucanase. At 48 hai, corresponding to the developmental stage where haustoria are produced by SR, many genes encoding proteins with a signal peptide were expressed. Haustoria are mostly responsible of nutrient uptake from the plant host, but it has also been identified as a site where fungal effectors proteins are secreted. Many other genes were expressed, but no known function was associated with them.

Table 1. Longest SR contigs expressed at 7, 24 and 48 hai, displaying similarity to proteins in different public databases and encoding signal peptides (SP)

Time-point[a]	Contig length[b]	Proteins	Organism	Evalue	SP
7	173	3-ketosteroid-delta-1-dehydrogenase	Magnaporthe grisea	0.017	Yes
	129	NA[c]	NA	NA	Yes
	122	unknown	Verticillium dahliae	0.012	No
	111	NA	NA	NA	Yes
	105	NA	NA	NA	Yes
	105	NADH-cytochrome b5 reductase	M. grisea	0.05	Yes
	103	60S ribosomal protein L10	Phytophtora sojae	0.095	Yes
	102	methylenetetrahydrofolate reductase	P. sojae	6E-04	Yes
24	127	unknown	Alternaria brassicicola	0.012	Yes
	119	NA	NA	NA	Yes
	113	unknown	Ophiostoma novo-ulmi	1E-05	Yes
	112	ABC transporter ATP-binding protein	P. sojae	0.011	Yes
	112	D-3-phosphoglycerate dehydrogenase	P. sojae	0.05	No
	106	unknown	O. novo-ulmi	3E-12	No
	106	beta-1,4-mannosyltransferase	P. sojae	0.069	Yes
	106	beta-1,3-glucanase	M. grisea	0.069	No
	104	carnitine/acylcarnitine translocase	P. sojae	0.046	No
	103	DHHC-type zinc finger domain-containing protein	P. sojae	0.099	Yes
	101	64 kDa mitochondrial NADH dehydrogenase	M. grisea	0.037	No
	101	uroporphyrinogen decarboxylase	M. grisae	0.037	Yes
	100	unknown	P. sojae	0.002	No
48	117	NA	NA	NA	Yes
	113	unknown	Blumeria graminis	4E-13	Yes
	112	sirodesmin biosynthesis protein	Leptosphaeria maculans	0.057	Yes

[a] Time-point expressed in hours after inoculation.
[b] Contig length in base pair.
[c] NA for not applicable.

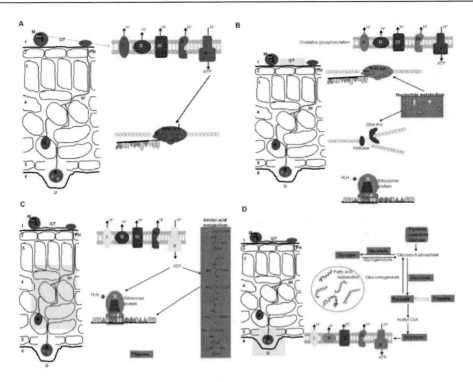

Figure 2. Schematic representation of events occurring in the pathogen during the infection process; (A) 15 sai; (B) 7 hai, (C) 48 hai, and (D) 10 dai of a susceptible soybean leaf with *Phakopsora pachyrhizi*. Drawing in black represents a cross-section of a soybean leaf where zone 1 represents the upper cuticle, zone 2 the upper epidermis cell layer, zone 3 the palisade mesophyll cell layer, zone 4 the spongy mesophyll cell layer, zone 5 the lower epidermis cell layer, and zone 6 the lower cuticle. Drawing in brown represents *P. pachyrhizi* structures on and inside the soybean leaf showing spore (S), mitochondrion (M), germ tube (GT), appressorium (A), primary hypha (PH), infectious hyphae (IH), haustorium (H), and uredinium (U). Highlight in yellow indicates where activities shown on the right side occur. Metabolic pathways, proteins, E. C. numbers, products, and substrates colored in blue are activated or expressed; those colored in green are up-regulated compared to the previous time-point; and those colored in red are down-regulated compared to the previous time-point; while boxes colored in yellow represent enzymes encoded by mRNAs with varied regulatory status. Metabolic pathways, proteins, E.C. numbers, products, and substrates colored in black were not activated or expressed in the present data set.

Taking into account the low number of genes that we identified using LCM samples, cDNA libraries were synthesized using RNA extracted from whole leaves of soybean cultivar Williams 82 fifteen seconds infection as well as 7, 48 and 240 hai. These time-points correspond to crucial steps into rust infection named pre-penetration, colonization, and sporulation stages. The resulting sequences were a combination of soybean and SR sequences.

The availability of the soybean genome provided an appropriate template to build contigs from the millions of sequences obtained by deep sequencing and, allowed easy identificaextraction of soybean genes from those million sequences. Those contiggenes not matching sequences from the soybean genome were considered as potentially from SR genes. Fifteen seconds after infection, 6,531 *de novo* transcripts were assembled from potential SR sequences. At 7, 48 and 240 hai, 4,627; 4,273 and; 12,284 *de novo* transcripts were assembled. In summary our study showed that energy production is highly active in ungerminated spores reflected by the abundant expression of mRNAs encoding complexes I,

IV, and V involved in oxidative phosphorylation and mRNAs encoding proteins involved in glycolysis such as phosphoglucomutase, fructose-1,6-bisphosphatase and triosephosphate isomerase. The energy produced by these metabolic pathways can be used by RNA polymerases.; mRNA for these wasere also highly expressed and the enzyme can transcribed genes necessary for the subsequent step of fungal growth. During the pre-penetration step, where spores are germinating, transcripts of genes encoding enzymes involved in nucleotide metabolism wasere an abundancet along with transcripts of genes encoding proteins involved in protein synthesis while genes encoding enzymes involved in energy production tended to be down-regulated. At 48 hai, haustoria developed in host cells as part of the colonization stage. At this specific time-point, there were an abundance of genes encoding enzymes involved in amino acid metabolism and protein synthesis supporting the recent hypothesis that haustoria play additional roles in addition to than only nutrient uptake. There were also a high number of mRNAs sharing similarity to genes encoding enzymes involved in lipid metabolism and carbohydrate metabolisms that may be associated with the synthesis and expansion of hyphal and haustorial walls and membranes. Finally, at the end of the infection process, transcripts of genes encoding enzymes involved in carbohydrate and fatty acid metabolism were the most highly abundant. Many genes encoding proteins involved in other metabolic pathways were expressidentified at this latest stage of infection and the complete study has been published by Tremblay et al., 2011. Our data also suggested that the thiamine metabolism is highly activated all along the infection process but specifically at 48 and 240 hai. However, there is no known physiological role associated with thiamine, but it seems to be important in *P. pachyrhizi* spore germination and during haustoria maturation through to the end of the infection process. Figure 2. illustrates the possible succession of events occurring in a susceptible soybean leaf over the time-course of infection with *P. pachyrhizi*.

Applications of Candidate Genes

Once genes are identified that are important to fungal germination, penetration, growth and reproduction, how can they be used to thwart the fungus? Likewise, once soybean genes are identified that are expressed in response to attack by SR in susceptible and resistant soybean leaves, how can this knowledge be used to develop soybean with resistance to the fungus? It may be possible to silence the fungal genes by having the soybean plant over-produce RNAi targeted against critical fungal genes. This can be explored using transgenic plants or through virus induced gene silencing (VIGS). Pandey et al. (2011) used VIGS to test 140 candidate genes for potential SR resistance mediated by *Rpp2*.

Eleven genes have been positively identified as required for *Rpp2*-mediated resistance against SR. Perhaps antibodies can be made against specific fungal proteins and can be expressed by the plant to inhibit their action. Over-expression of specific soybean genes involved in signaling and the defense response could be viable strategy as well. Or perhaps suppression of other soybean genes may decrease the likelihood of survival of the rust.

Conclusion

Considering the little information we have on fungi development and plant-fungi interactions in general and the big concern about field losses due to plant fungi, the emergence of new technologies opens new ways to explore and find strategies to decrease or completely eradicate some plants fungali infections, such as soybean rust.

Acknowledgments

The authors thank Leslie Wanner for her careful critical review of the manuscript. Mention of trade names or commercial products in this article is solely for the purpose of providing specific information and does not imply recommendation or endorsement by the United States Department of Agriculture.

References

Asano T, Masumura T, Kusano H, Kikuchi S, Kurita A, Shimada H, Kadowaki K (2002) Construction of a specialized cDNA library from plant cells isolated by laser capture microdissection: Toward comprehensive analysis of the genes expressed in the rice phloem. *The Plant Journal* 32, 401-408.

Bennett S (2004) Solexa Ltd. *Pharmacogenomics* 5, 433-438.

Bennett ST, Barnes C, Cox A, Davies L, Brown C (2005) Toward the $1000 human genome. *Pharmacogenomics* 6, 373-382.

Burgoon MP, Keays KM, Owens GP, Ritchie AM, Rai PR, Cool CD, Gilden DH (2005) Laser-capture microdissection of plasma cells from subacute sclerosing panencephalitis brain reveals intrathecal disease-relevant antibodies. *Proceedings of the National Academy of Sciences USA* 102, 7245-7250.

Choi JJ, Alkharouf NW, Schneider KT, Matthews BF, Frederick RD (2008) An enriched cDNA library and microarray analysis reveal expression patterns in soybean resistant to soybean rust. *Functional and Integrative Genomics* 8, 341-351.

Curran S, Murray GI (2005) An introduction to laser-based tissue microdissection techniques. *Methods in Molecular Biology* 293, 3-8.

Denoeud F, Aury J-M, da Silva C, Noel B, Rogier O, Delledonne M, Morgante M, Valle G, Wincker P, Scarpelli C, Jaillon O, Artiguenave F (2008) Annotating genomes with massive-scale RNA sequencing. *Genome Biology* 9, R175.

Emmert-Buck MR, Bonner RF, Smith PD, Chauqui RF, Zhuang Z, Goldstein SR, Weiss RA, Liotta LA (1996) Laser capture microdissection. *Science* 274, 998-1001.

Garcia A, Calvo ÉS, de Souza Kiihl RA, Harada A, Hiromoto DM, Vieira LGE (2008) Molecular mapping of soybean rust (*Phakopsora pachyrhizi*) resistance genes: discovery of a novel locus and alleles. *Theoretical and Applied Genetics* 117, 545-553.

Hacquard S, Delaruelle C, Legué V, Tisserant E, Kohler A, Frey P, Martin F, Duplessis S (2010) Laser capture microdissection of uredinia formed by *Melampsora larici-populina* revealed a transcriptional switch between biotrophy and sporulation. *Molecular Plant-Microbe Interactions* 23, 1275-1286.

Hahn M, Mendgen K (1997) Characterization of *in planta*–induced rust genes isolated from a haustorium-specific cDNA library. *Molecular Plant-Microbe Interaction* 10, 427-437.

Herzenberg LA, Parks D, Sahaf B, Perez O, Roederer M, Herzenberg LA (2002) The history and future of the fluorescence activated cell sorter and flow cytometry: A view from Stanford. *Clinical Chemistry* 48, 1819-1827.

Kerk NM, Ceserani T, Tausta SL, Sussex IM, Nelson TM (2003) Laser capture microdissection of cells from plant tissues. *Plant Physiology* 132, 27-35.

Klink, V., M.H. MacDonald and B.F. Matthews (2005) Gene expression in soybean syncytial cells formed by the soybean cyst nematode and isolated by laser-capture microdissection. *Plant Molecular Biology* 59, 969-983.

Klink, V.P., C.C. Overall, N.W. Alkharouf, M.H. MacDonald, B.F. Matthews (2007) Laser capture microdissection (LCM) and comparative microarray expression analysis of syncytial cells isolated from incompatible and compatible soybean roots infected by soybean cyst nematode (*Heterodera glycines*). *Planta* 226, 1389-1409.

Klink, V.P., P. Hosseini, P. Matsye, N.W. Alkharouf, B.F. Matthews (2009) A gene expression analysis of syncytia laser microdissected from the roots of the *Glycine max* (soybean) genotype PI 548402 (Peking) undergoing a resistant reaction after infection by *Heterodera glycines* (soybean cyst nematode). *Plant Molecular Biology* 71, 525-567.

Klink, V.P., P. Hosseini, P. Matsye, N.W. Alkharouf, B.F. Matthews (2010a) Syncytium gene expression in *Glycine ma* [PI 88788] roots undergoing a resistant reaction to the parasitic nematode *Heterodera glycines*. *Plant Physiology and Biochemistry* 48, 176-193.

Klink, V.P., C.C. Overall, N.W. Alkharouf, M.H. MacDonald, B.F. Matthews (2010b) Microarray detection calls as a means to compare transcripts expressed within syncytial cells isolated from incompatible and compatible soybean (Glycine max) roots infected by the soybean cyst nematode (Heterodera glycines). *Journal of Biomedicine and Biotechnology* 1-30.

Klink, V.P., P. Hosseini, P. Matsye, N.W. Alkharouf, B.F. Matthews (2011) Differences in gene expression amplitude overlie a conserved transcriptomic program occurring between the rapid and potent localized resistant reaction at the syncytium of the *Glycine max* genotype Peking (PI 548402) as compared to the prolonged and potent resistant reaction of PI 88788. *Plant Molecular Biology* 75, 141-165.

Liszewski K (2007) Laser-capture microdissection advances. Point-and-shoot technology makes isolating pure cell populations almost a breeze. *Genetic Engineering and Biotechnology News* 27 (2).

Miles MR, Frederick RD, Hartman GL (2006) Evaluation of soybean germplasm for resistance to *Phakopsora pachyrhizi*. *Plant Health Progress* Doi:10.1094/PHP-2006-0104-01-RS.

Miles MR, Morel W, Ray JD, Smith JR, Frederick RD, Hartman GL (2008) Adult plant evaluation of soybean accessions for resistance to *Phakopsora pachyrhizi* in the field and greenhouse in Paraguay. *Plant Disease* 92, 96-105.

Margulies M, Egholm M, Altman WE, Attiya S, Bader JS, Bemben LA, Berka J, Braverman MS, Chen Y-J, Chen Z, Dewell SB, Du L, Fierro JM, Gomes XV, Godwin BC, He W, Helgesen S, Ho CH, Irzyk GP, Jando SC, Alenquer MLI, Jarvie TP, Jirage KB, Kim J-B, Knight JR, Lanza JR, Leamon JH, Lefkowitz SM, Lei M, Li J, Lohman KL, Lu H,

Makhijani VB, McDade KE, McKenna MP, Myers EW, Nickerson E, Nobile JR, Plant R, Puc BP, Ronan MT, Roth GT, Sarkis GJ, Simons JF, Simpson JW, Srinivasan M, Tartaro KR, Tomasz A, Vogt KA, Volkmer GA, Wang SH, Wang Y, Weiner MP, Yu P, Begley RF, Rothberg JM (2005) Genome sequencing in microfabricated high-density picolitre reactors *Nature* 437, 376-380.

Nakazono M, Qui F, Borsuk LA, Schnable PS (2003) Laser-capture microdissection, a tool for the global analysis of gene expression in specific plant cell types: Identification of genes expressed differentially in epidermal cells or vascular tissues of maize. *The Plant Cell* 15, 583-596

Pandey AK, Yang C, Zhang C, Graham MA, Horstman HD, Lee Y, Zabotina OA, Hill JH, Pedley KF, Whitham SA (2011) Functional analysis of the Asian soybean rust resistance pathway mediated by *Rpp2*. *Molecular Plant-Microbe Interactions* 24, 194-206.

Panthee, DR, Yuan JS, Wright DL, Marois JJ, Mailhot D, Stewart Jr. CN (2006) Gene expression analysis in soybean in response to the causal agent of Asian soybean rust (*Phakopsora pachyrhizi* Sydow) in an early growth stage. *Functional Integrated Genomics* 7, 291-301.

Panthee DR, Marois JJ, Wright DL, Narváez D, Yuan JS, Stewart Jr. CN (2009) Differential expression of genes in soybean in response to the causal agent of Asian soybean rust (*Phakopsora pachyrhizi* Sydow) is soybean growth stage-specific. *Theoretical and Applied Genetics* 118, 359-370.

Peterson LA, Brown MR, Carlisle AJ, Kohn EC, Liotta LA, Emmert-Buck MR, Krizman DB (1998) An improved method for construction of directionally cloned cDNA libraries from microdissected cells. *Cancer Research* 58, 5326–5328.

Posada-Buitrago ML, Frederick RD (2005) Expressed sequence tag analysis of the soybean rust pathogen *Phakopsora pachyrhizi*. *Fungal Genetics and Biology* 42, 949-962.

Ronaghi M (2001) Pyrosequencing sheds light on DNA sequencing. Genome Research 11, 3-11.

Simone NL, Bonner RF, Gillespie JW, Emmert-Buck MR, Liotta LA (1998) Laser-capture microdissection: opening the microscopic frontier to molecular analysis. *Trends in Genetics* 14, 272-276.

Soria-Guerra RE, Rosales-Mendoza S, Chang S, Haudenshield JS, Padmanaban A, Rodriguez-Zas S, Hartman GL, Ghabrial SA, Korban SS (2009) Transciptome analysis of resistant and susceptible genotypes of *Glycine tomentella* during *Phakopsora pachyrhizi* infection reveals novel rust resistance genes. *Theoretical and applied Genetics* 120, 1315-1333.

Sanger F, Nicklen S, Coulson AR (1977) DNA sequencing with chain-terminating inhibitors. *Proceedings of the National Academy of Sciences USA* 74, 5463-5467.

Tiburzi R, Martins EMF, Reisener HJ (1992) Isolation of haustoria of *Puccinia graminis f. sp. tritici* from wheat leaves. *Experimental Mycology* 16, 324-328.

Tremblay A, Li S, Scheffler BE, Matthews BF (2008) Laser capture microdissection and expressed sequence tag analysis of uredinia formed by *Phakopsora pachyrhizi,* the causal agent of soybean rust. *Physiological and Molecular Plant Pathology* 73, 163-174.

Tremblay A, Hosseini P, Alkharouf NW, Li S, Matthews BF (2010) Transcriptome analysis of a compatible response by *Glycine max* to *Phakopsora pachyrhizi* infection. *Plant Science* 179, 183-193.

Tremblay A, Hosseini P, Li S, Alkharouf NW, Matthews BF (2011) Identification of genes expressed by *Phakopsora pachyrhizi*, the pathogen causing soybean rust, at a late stage of infection of susceptible soybean leaves. *Plant Pathology* 61, 773-786.

van de Mortel M, Recknor R, Graham MA, Nettleton D, Dittman JD, Nelson RT, Godoy CV, Abdelnoor RV, Almeida AMR, Baum TJ, Whitham SA (2007) Distinct biphasic mRNA changes in response to Asian soybean rust infection. *Molecular Plant-Microbe Interactions* 20, 887-899.

Wong MH, Saam JR, Stappenbeck TS, Rexer CH, Gordon JI (2000) Genetic mosaic analysis based on *Cre* recombinase and navigated laser capture microdissection. *Proceedings of the National Academy of Sciences USA* 97, 12601-12606.

Yang S-Y, Lien K-Y, Huang K-J, Lei H-Y, Lee G-B (2008) Micro flow cytometry utilizing a magnetic bead-based immunoassay for rapid virus detection. *Biosensors and Bioelectronics* 24, 855-862.

Yorinori JT, Paiva WM, Frederick RD, Costamilan LM, Bertagnolli PF, Hartman GE, Godoy CV, Nunes Jr. J (2005) Epidemics of soybean rust (*Phakopsora pachyrhizi*) in Brazil and Paraguay from 2001 to 2003. *Plant Disease* 89, 675-677.

In: Advances in Medicine and Biology. Volume 69   ISBN: 978-1-62808-088-9
Editor: Leon V. Berhardt   © 2013 Nova Science Publishers, Inc.

Chapter V

Diversity and Evolution of Fungal Phytopathogens Associated with Snow

***Tamotsu Hoshino[1, 2]*, Yuka Yajima[1], Oleg B. Tkachenko[3],
Yousuke Degawa[4], Motoaki Tojo[5] and Naoyuki Matsumoto[6]***

[1]National Institute of Advanced Industrial Science and Technology (AIST),
Higashi-Hiroshima, Japan
[2]Graduate School of Life Science, Hokkaido University, Sapporo, Japan
[3]Main Botanical Garden, Russian Academy of Sciences, Moscow, Russia
[4]Sugadaira Montane Research Center, University of Tsukuba, Ueda, Japan
[5]Graduate School of Life and Environmental Sciences,
Osaka Prefecture University, Sakai, Japan
[6]Graduate School of Agriculture, Hokkaido University, Sapporo, Japan

Abstract

Cryophilic fungi spend a certain life stage or whole life cycle (sexual and/or asexual reproduction) in the cryosphere where biosphere is constantly or seasonally covered with snow and/or ice. Several groups of cryophilic fungi and their relatives infect other living organisms including fungi. Cryophilic fungal phytopathogens exist in different depths of snow cover, according to their ecophysiological characteristics. Snow fungi represent a fungal group growing on the snow surface, consisting of chytridiomycetes and ascomycete. They are pathogenic to algae growing on the snow. Chytridiomycetes have flagella in a certain stage of their life cycles to reach and infect their hosts, inciting diseases on algae. Snow molds attack overwintering plants within and under snow and include various fungal taxa (mainly oomycetes, ascomycetes and basidiomycetes).

* Corresponding author: Tamotsu Hoshino (e-mail: tamotsu.hoshino@aist.go.jp)

Ascomycetous snow molds are pathogenic on the needles of conifers, causing defoliation and blight in snow. They are adapted to xeric conditions and infect hard host tissues such as conifer needles. Herbaceous plants are attacked by a variety of cryophilic fungal phytopathogens under snow where antagonism from mesophilic microorganisms seldom occurs. These fungi are well adapted to the environment where ambient temperature vary at around subzero temperatures. Cyst-like fungal bodies are observed inside fruit bodies of snowbank slime molds (nivicolous myxomycetes). Phylogenetic analyses suggested that they belonged to cryptomycota. In conclusion, cryophilic pathogens are evolved from diverse fungal taxa to adapt to nival environments, developing cold tolerance and selecting host organisms.

Introduction

Approximately 80% of the biosphere is constantly or seasonally cold and has temperatures below 5°C [e.g. 1]. The biosphere, with an exception of deep sea, is almost identical to the cryosphere. The term cryosphere was proposed by the Polish scientist, A.B. Dobrowolski and collectively describes the portions of the Earth's surface where water exists as the frozen state - snow cover, glaciers, ice sheets and shelves, freshwater ice, sea ice, icebergs, permafrost, and ground ice [2]. The cryosphere creates a seasonally extreme environment in temperate and frigid zones and often disappears in summer. Fungi associated with seasonal snow, ice and frozen, ground, so far termed as psychrophiles [3], should adapt to a wide temperature range from subzero temperatures to over 20°C , i.e., their maximal growth temperature.

Fungal species were less frequently recorded from the cryosphere than those of temperate zone despite that major fungal taxa have already been found in the cryosphere [4, 5]. These records suggest a possibility that various fungi are active under diverse cold environments. Fungi normally have different cells in their life cycle; fungal thermal dependence varies according to their life cycle stages and is completely different from that of bacteria.

Examples are illustrated to show that the concept of psychrophile in bacteria by Morita [3] does not apply to fungi, and we proposed a new term "cryophilic fungi" for those that spend a certain life stage or whole life cycle (sexual and/or asexual reproduction) in the cryosphere [5].

According to sexual reproduction, the true fungi were divided into 4 phyla (Chytridiomycota, traditional Zygomycota, Ascomycota and Basidiomycota). Though recent phylogenetic analysis revealed that fungi are composed of 7 phyla and uncertain 4 subphyla [6], we will use the former 4 phyla in this review. Cryophilic fungi include not only saprophytes but also parasites, as well as symbionts [4, 5]. Some groups of cryophilic fungi attack overwintering plants and other living organisms including fungi on/in/under snow. In this review, we discuss the diversity and ecophysiological characteristics of these fungi.

Pathogenic Fungi on Snow

The cryoseston is defined as the community of organisms living on snow [7]. Algae grow on snow and named "snow algae". Snow algae are major organisms in the cryoseston, and fungi that associate with snow algae are referred to as snow fungi. Kol [8, 9] listed 82 species of snow fungi including 3 fungal pathogens of snow algae, i.e., the chytridiomycetes *Chytridium chlamydococci* f. *cryophila* (Nom. Inval.), *Rhizophydium sphaerocarpum* subsp. *cryophilum* and the ascomycete *Oospora nivalis* [8, 10].

C. *chlamydococci* f. *cryophila* was recovered in the cells of algae, *Chlamidomonas bolyaiana* in South America, *C. nivalis* in several areas in Europe, *C. sangunea* in Romania and *Ancylonema nordenskoiöldii* in Greenland [8]. *R. sphaerocarpum* subsp. *cryophilum* was found in the cells of *A. nordenskoiöldii* in Alaska [8, 11]. *Rhizophydium* sp. often attached *Chlamydomonas* sp. in Colorado [12]. *Oospora nivalis* coexisted with *C. nivalis* but its pathogenicity was not unambiguously described [10]. Kobayashi and Ôkubo also reported that *Chytridium neochlamydococci* and *Rhizophydium* sp. in cells of the snow alga, *C. nivalis* in Ozegahara, Japan [13, 14].

Snow algae, the hosts of fungal pathogens, are mostly flagellate. Their resting spores germinate in the soil under snow, and flagellated cells swim upward through the thaw water surrounding snow crystals until they reach the surface of snowpack [15]. The chytridiomycetes represent a dominant fungal group under the snow cover [16, 17] and are typical algal pathogens in water-ecosystems [18].

These fungi also have flagella in their life cycles [18]. Their life cycle is shown in Figure 1A. With the onset of spring, melting snow adds nutrients to freshwater lakes, and the rise in temperature facilitates the rapid growth of algal phytoplankton. Soon after the algal bloom begins, the growth of parasitic zoosporic true fungi causes "chytrid epidemic" [18, 19]. Chytrid epidemic may also occur on the snow based on the similar mechanism.

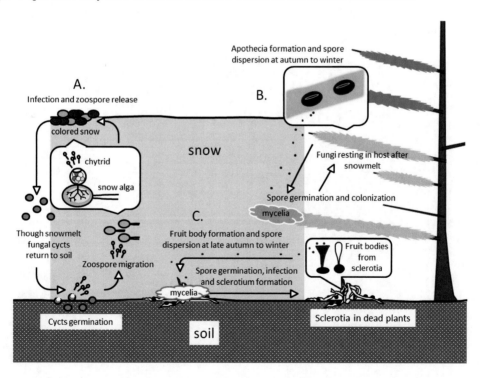

Figure 1. Life cycles of cryophilic fungal phytopathogens associated with snow. A. snow fungi (chytridiomycetes) in winter to spring. B. snow blight fungi (e.g., *Phacidium infestans*) in autumn to winter. C. snow molds (*Sclerotinia borealis* and *Typhula ishikariensis*) in autumn to winter.

Pathogenic Fungi within Snow

Snow blight is cryophilic fungal diseases of conifers [e.g. 20, 21]. Withered needles below the snowline are matted together with grayish or black brown mycelia and infected seedlings occur in patches. These fungal pathogens are exclusively ascomycetes such as *Hemiphacidium convexum*, *Herpotrichia coulteri*, *Herpotrichia juniper*, *Herpotrichia nigra*, *Lophophacidium hyperboreum*, *Neopeckia coulteri*, *Nothophacidium abietinellum*, *Sarcotrochila balsameae*, *Sarcotrochila piniperda*, *Phacidium abietis* (basionym: *P. infectans* var. *abietis*), *Phacidium infestans* (syn. *Phacidium abietis*, including 2 forma and 3 varieties) and *Phacidium taxicola* [21−24]. *L. hyperboreum*, *P. abietis* and *P. infestans* infect needles in the autumn via ascospores and remain latent until plants are covered with snow. Apothecia continue to release spores at temperatures around 0°C [25−27]. *P. infestans* can spread from branch to branch in snow [28, 29]. Their life cycle was shown in Figure 1B.

Mesophilic ascomycetes *Gremmeniella abietina* var. *abietina* and *G. abietina* var. *balsamea* cause scleroderris canker of conifers [29]. Plants with diseased needles are often found below the snowline, and winter temperatures influence infection rate; those overwintering at -7 and -3°C were more seriously diseased than those kept at 0°C [30]. These fungi can grow at subzero temperatures [31]. These findings suggest that *G. abietina* is active in a wide temperature range between subzero to summer air temperatures in the cryosphere. Similar life cycle occurs in the ascomycete *Microsphaeropsis* sp., causing canker on *Cornus controversa* [32]. Fungi capable of attack on woody plants in snow exhibit physiological characteristics as follows. 1) Adaptation to xeric. Causal fungi of snow blight and scleroderris canker do not require so much water for colonization in snow as do chytridiomyceteous snow fungi to swim in thaw water on snow surface, using flagella.

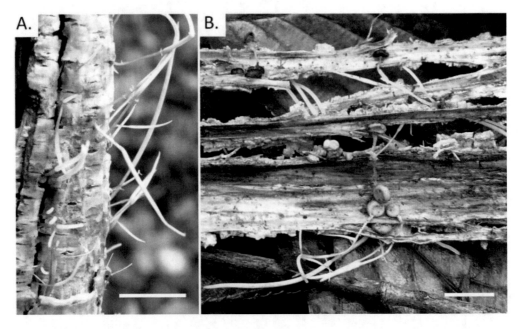

Figure 2. Basidiocarps of saprophytic *Typhula* spp. on the bark of *Euonymus alatus* f. *ciliatodentaus* on Sugadaira, Nagano, Japan (Hoshino et al., unpublished). A. basidiocarps on decayed bark, B. sclerotia on the inside of the bark. Both bars are 1 cm.

These ascomycetous pathogens are filamentous and can spread by extending hyphae. 2) Usage of hardy substrate in nutrient-depleted environment. Some of ascomycetous cryophilic phytopathogens use hard substrate of conifer needles. A fungus, believed to be *Phacidium infestans* extend web-like mycelia over the surface of snowbank during snowmelt [15]. Cells of snow algae, *Chloromonas cryophila* [33] and *Chloromonas pinchichae* [34] are frequency found adhered to the surface of the fungal mucelia, but there is no evidence of symbiosis as is found in lichens. Possibly, the fungus and algae may exchange metabolites extracellularly. Microscopic characterization is, unfortunately, not available on the web-like fungus.

Basidiomycete, *Typhula* is typical cryophilic pathogen under the snow and not in the snow. However saprophytic species of this genus was present on a bark of *Euonymus alatus* f. *ciliatodentaus* (Figure 2). In the cryosphere, known ascomycetes are ca. 1.6−5.8 times greater in number than basidiomycetes [4]. Ascomycetous cryophilic phytopatogens are higher diversity than those of other taxa.

Pathogenic Fungi under Snow

Snow molds are cryophilic fungal pathogens of forage crops, winter cereals, and conifers [e.g. 20, 24, 35, 36]. These fungi can attack dormant plants at low temperatures under snow. Snow cover protects overwintering plants from freezing and maintains darkness, humidity, and low temperature, which, as described in detail by Matsumoto and Hoshino [36], characterize the nature of snow molds as opportunistic pathogens. "Snow molds" or "snow mold fungi" is a generic name including diverse fungi in temperate to fridge zones belonging to various taxa i.e., oomycetes, ascomycetes, and basidiomycetes), but chytridiomycetes or traditional zygomycetes are not included.

Snow molds of agricultural crops are as follows (important pathogens are shown in bold letters) [24, 35, 37, 38]. Oomycetes: *Pythium iwayamai*, *Pythium okanoganense*, *Pythium paddicum*, *Pythium ultimum*, *Pythium volutum*; ascomycetes: *Dactylaria graminicola*, *Didymella pheina* (syn.: *Ascochyta phleina*), *Epicoccum nigrum* (syn.: *Epicoccum purpurascens*), *Gibberella avenacea* (syn.: *Fusarium avenaceum*), *Monographella nivalis* var. *nivalis* (syn.: *Microdochium nivale* var. *nivale*), *Microdochium nivale* var. *majus*, *Nectria tuberculariformis* (Anamorph: *Acremonium boreale* [35]), *Phoma sclerotioides* (syn.: *Plenodomus meliloti* [35]), *Sclerotinia borealis* (syn.: *Myriosclerotinia borealis*), *Sclerotinia nivalis*, *Sclerotinia trifoliorum*; basidiomycetes: *Atheria* sp. in Hokkaido, Japan [24], *Ceratobasidium gramineum*, *Coprinus psychromorbidus* in North America, *Rhizoctonia* sp. in Alberta, Canada [35], *Laetisaria fuciformis* (syn.: *Corticium fuciforme*), *Typhula incarnata*, *Typhula ishikariensis* var. *ishikariensis* (syn.: *Typhula borealis*, *Typhula hyperborea*), *T. ishikariensis* var. *idahoensis* (syn.: *Typhula idahoensis*), *T. ishikariensis* var. *canadiensis*, *Typhula japonica* in Japan [39], *Typhula phacorrhiza*, *Typhula trifolii*, *Typhula variabilis*; incertae sedis: *Sclerotium nivale* (Nom. Inval.) in Russia [38], *Sclerotium rhizodes*.

Snow molds of conifer seedlings are mostly ascomycetes [24, 40, 41] such as *Botrytis cinerea*, *Cylindrocarpon* sp. in Japan, *Racodium therryanum* in Asia, *S. borealis* (syn. *S. graminearum*) in Volga-Ural, Russia, *Sclerotinia kitajimana* in Japan, and previously described conifer pathogens in snow. Few basidiomycetes are known as conifer snow molds such as *Thanatephorus cucumeris* (syn.: *Rhizoctonia solani*) in Japan [40], *T. ishikariensis* (syn.: *Typhula graminearum* [Nom. Inval.]) in Volga-Ural, Russia [41], as well as incertae sedis: *Sclerotium* sp. (Ezo-raigan disease, non. *Agrocybe tuberosa*) in Hokkaido, Japan [40]. Basidiomycete *Cylindrobasidium parasiticum* is a mycoparasite of sclerotia of *T. incarnata* in Scotland [42], and ascomycetes *Episclerotium sclerotium* and *Episclerotium sclerotipus* are also [43] parasites of sclerotia of *T. phacorrhiza* and *Sclerotinia* spp.

The presence of a novel fungal structure has recently been found from myxomycetes under snow [44]. Cyst-like fungal bodies were present in the sporophores of nivicolous myxomycetes *Lamproderma* sp. and *Lamproderma* echinosporum (Figure 3). Numerous cyst-like fungal bodies were observed inside developing spores, capillitium, columella and stalk. They were transparent, spherical 5−6 μm in diameter, warted had spines. Partial sequences of 18S rDNA gene from infected *Lamproderma* sp. contained a novel sequence, suggesting that cyst-like fungal bodies belonged to the Cryptomycota [45] positioned at the root of a fungal clade. Since Cryptomycota can be phagotrophic parasites, the behavior of the cyst-like fungal bodies should be further studies elucidate to host-parasite interactions under snow.

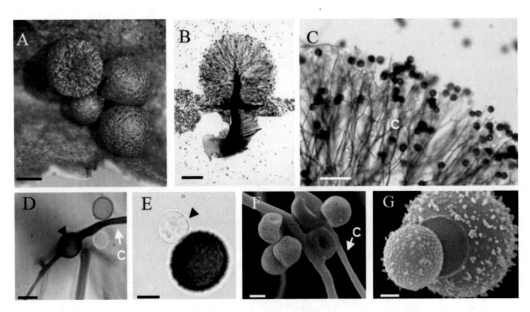

Figure 3. Cyst-like fungal bodies are observed inside of fruit bodies of snowbank slime mold. A: sporophores of *Lamproderma echinosporum,* TNS-M-H 7200. One of the sporocarps showing many white grains (fungal cyst-like bodies) inside the sporophore. B-E. light micrographs of *L. echinosporum* with fungal cyst-like bodies. B: sporophore. C: tip of capillitium (C). D: part of capillitum with two cyst-like bodies. E: a spore and a invading cyst-like body (arrow head). F, G: scanning electron micrographs of *L. echinosporum* with fungal cyst-like bodies. F: part of capillitium and 6 fungal cyst-like bodies. G: a spore and a fungal cyst-like body. Bars in: A:1mm, B: 0.3mm, C: 100μm, D, E: 5μm, F, G: 2μm.

Snow molds have different adaptation strategies against freezing stress [46]. Oomycetes, *Pythium* spp. were reported to be less tolerant to chilling and freezing temperatures than other fungal taxa [47−49]. Free mycelia and hyphal swellings, structures for survival, of *P. iwayamai* lost viability after cycles of freezing-thawing. However mycelia in host plants survived the treatment [4, 46]. Basidiomycetous snow molds produce extracellular antifreeze proteins which attach to the surface of ice crystal to inhibit ice crystal growth [24, 50]. An ascomycete, *Sclerotinia borealis* prevails where soil freezing is severe. Mycelial growth on frozen plates at -1°C was faster than that on unfrozen medium at the optimal growth temperature of 4−10°C [24, 51]. *S. borealis* can grow at low water potential on media, and an increase in intracellular osmosis enhances mycelial growth at low temperatures. Though, as a whole, snow mold can tolerate low temperatures to prevail under snow, survival strategies to adapt in the cryosphere differ from fungus to fungus, according to the preference in their particular habitats.

Fungi show the highest diversity along the vertical section of snow, interacting other microbes and plants under snow. Wolf and Wolf [52] stated that conceivably, the temperature differential might be an important factor when two or more species were competing for substrata but that it may not necessarily constitute the controlling factor. Pathogenic activity of *P. infestans* fungus in the snow is influenced by ground vegetation [23], and the fungus spread rapidly in pine-*Cladonia* forests types, where vegetation on the ground is very poor. Healthy and dead foliage inhibited spread of *P. infestans* [53].

Mycelial growth of *T. ishikariensis* var. *ishikariensis* on potato dextrose agar at 0°C was half that of its optimal growth at 10°C. However, when cultures were covered with unsterile soil to introduce natural microbial antagonists, mycelial growth was much less at 10°C than at 0°C [54, 55]. These facts indicate that *T. ishikariensis* var. *ishikariensis* is unable to develop mycelia at 10°C in nature, and this fungus prevails at subzero temperatures where microbial antagonists are not active.

Pathogenic Fungi in Soil under Snow

Some species of snow molds are soilborne pathogens and cause disease on underground parts of overwintering plants [38, 41, 56]. Ascomycetes: *S. borealis* in Alaska [57], *S. kitajimana*, *R. therryanum*; basidiomycetes: *T. incarnata* [58], *T. ishikariensis* var. *ishikariensis* in Russia [38, 41]; incertae sedis: *Sclerotium* sp. in Hokkaido, Japan [59]. Soil microbes affect the survival of fungal sclerotia, and sclerotium-forming fungi have two ways to avoid microbial contaminations in their sclerotia, secretion of antibiotics and secondary sclerotium formation [60, 61]. Small, secondary sclerotia of snow molds were first found within sclerotia of *T. ishikariensis* var. *idahoensis* placed on moist sand for 90 day [62]. Sclerotia of *T. ishikariensis* var. *idahoensis* were more effective in inciting snow molds of winter wheat when placed on the soil surface than when buried 0.5 or 1.0 cm in soil, and were not effective when buried 2 to 10 cm in soil [62]. However, *T. ishikariensis* var. *ishikariensis* (syn.: *Typhula humlina*) causes diseases on tulip bulbs and hop roots in European part of Russia and Volga-Ural, Russia [38, 41]. *T. ishikariensis* var. *ishikariensis* in Russia can survive at a depth of 20 cm in soil for 13 months by forming secondary sclerotia [61, 63]. These ecophysiological characteristics are important for sclerotium survival of *T. ishikariensis* in Russia as a soilborn pathogen.

Snow Molds in Polar Regions

P. iwayamai has not been so far found in the Arctic or Antarctica, however a new heterothallic species, *Pythium polare* was isolated from moribund tissues of polar mosses in both poles [64]. Symptom on mosses caused by *P. polare* was the same [65, 66], and isolates from both poles were sexually compatible. The fungus was similar to *P. iwayamai* in ITS regions [64−66]. Sclerotium-forming snow molds *S. borealis*, *T. incarnata* and *T.*

ishikariensis are widely distributed in not only the cool temperate zone to frigid zone but also Arctic regions [65] such as Alaska and the Yukon [67], Greenland [68], Finnmark (northern Norway [37]), Iceland (*S. borealis* not found [69]), Lapland (northern Finland and Sweden: [70−72]), Kola Peninsula in the European part of Russia [73], Novaya Zemlya (*T. incarnata* found [74]) and Svalbard [75, 76]. Their distribution pattern suggests that *S. borealis* and *T. ishikariensis* are highly adapted to the Arctic environment. *S. borealis* and *T. ishikariensis* were not found from Antarctica. However, *Sclerotinia antarctica* on Antarctic hair grass *Deschampsia antarctica* was found in Antarctic peninsula. The fungus is morphological similar to *S. borealis* [77] and needs comparisons with *S. borealis*. We also found another fungal disease on the moss, *Polytrichum juniperium* on King George Island, Antarctica [4]. Sclerotia were not found on diseased plants; however, molecular data suggested that *Typhula* sp. was present there. These findings suggest that three genera of representative snow molds *Pyhtium*, *Sclerotinia* and *Typhula* could share the same niches in both polar regions.

Other fungal species are also recognized as snow molds in both poles [65]. Though usually regard as a saprobe in temperate zone, an ascomycete *Trichoderma polysporum* (teleomorph: *Hypocrea pachybasioides*) caused asympomatic infections on the moss *Sanionia uncinata* on Svalbard [78]. Basidiomycetous *Microbotryum bistortarum*, the smut fungus, was also shown to have deleterious effects on the growth and survival of Alpine Bistort *Polygonum vivparum* under snow cover also on Svalbard [79]. This fungus has similar life cycle of scleroderris canker disease fungus *Gremmeniella abietina*. Zygomycetous snow molds are not found in the Northern Hemisphere, but *Rhizopus* sp. was pathogen on the moss *Bryum anatrcticum* at Cape Bird on Ross Island [80]. Unfortunately, the specimens are not available (L. Greenfield, personal communication). Several ascomycetes *Thyronectria antarctica* var. *hyperantarctica*, *Coleroa turfosorum*, *Bryosphaeria megaspora*, *Epibryon chorisodontii* and an unidentified Plectomycete were recorded from ring infection and macroscopic section of mosses [81−83]. Cryophilic fungi are less in the number of species than that of fungi in temperate region [4], and flora in polar regions are different from other regions of cryosphere in temperate and frigid zones. Therefore, there must be new niches for cryophilic fungal phytopathogens in polar regions, and novel cryophilic fungi are likely to have evolved as phytopathogens to adapted in polar climate and vegetation.

Evolution of Cryophilic Fungal Phytopathogens

Fungal fossil diversity increased throughout the Paleozoic Era with all modern classes reported in the Pennsylvanian Epoch (320-286 Ma) [84]. Present climatic zones on earth were formed from the Cretaceous period (145-66 Ma), then plants adapted in cold environment [85]. Cryophilic fungal saprophytes probably also occurred from mesophilic saprophytes, and consequently some species of cryophilic fungi acquired pathogenicity against overwintering plants [86]. *Pythium*, *Sclerotinia* and *Typhula* are typical genera of snow molds, and species of mesophiles and psychrotolerants are greater in number than psychrophiles. Pathogenicity and cold-adaptation are essential factors for fungi to become cryophilic fungal phytopathogens, and these factors co-evolved in *Typhula* [87].

Pathogenicity is strongly correlated with freezing resistance in oomycetous snow molds [4, 46]. Fungi in permafrost are characterized by both the presence of natural cryoprotectants such as plant substrates or derivatives in these ecotopes and the ability to utilize their inherent mechanisms of protection [88]. Stakhov et al. [89] demonstrated that ancient seeds of higher plants constituted a specific habitat for microorganisms in frozen ground, which favored their survival for millennia. Cold-accumulated plants also store cryoprotectants in their cytosol, and *Pythium* spp. in infected tissues, probably utilize host cryoprotectants to tolerate freezing.

Snow mold are invariably stress tolerant, but their level of tolerance differs from fungus to fugus. They are either airborne or soilbore, or both. Airborne pathogens are ruderal or *r*-selected, reaching new habitat through spores before snow cover, and different strains of the same species share plant tissues to develop. Though not airborne, *Pythium* spp. have the same strategy. Soilborne snow molds, except *Pythium* spp., exploit plant tissues nearby and excludes other strains through intraspecific antagonism. *Typhula ishikariensis* is, in this context, a typical *K*-strategist among snow mold fungi [90]. The mode of epidemiology does not coincide with cold-tolerance in snow mold fungi and divide them into two categories, i.e., facaltative and obligate snow molds [91]. *Sclerotinia borealis*, *T. incarnata* and *T. ishikariensis* are obligate snow molds that prevail exclusively under snow and tolerant to cold with different mechanisms. *Pythium* spp. and *Microdochium nivale* are facaltative snow molds and can develop without snow even in summer when it is cool and damp. They are moderately tolerant to cold. Though fungal pathogens are less frequently recorded from the cryosphere than those from the temperate zone, their diversity in adaptation strategy is considerably high and needs further investigations to reveal the complex ecosystem of the cryosphere.

Conclusion

We described the diversity of cryophilic fungal phytopathogens and their environmental adaptations. Their diversity and ecophisiological characteristics vary along the vertical section of snow cover. Mesophilic saprophytes are considered to have become cryophilic saprophytes to adapt in cold environment, and then evolved into cryophilic phytopathogens, acquiring pathogenicity to overwintering plants.

References

[1]   Gounot, A.M. (1999). Microbial life in permanently cold soils. In: Margesin, R. and Schinner, F., editors. *Cold-adapted organisms: Ecology, physiology, enzymology and molecular biology.* Berlin: Springer ; pp. 3−16.

[2]   Barry, R. and Gan, T.Y. (2011). *The Global Cryosphere Past, Present and Future.* Cambridge: Cambridge University Press.

[3]   Morita, R.Y. (1975). Psychrophilic bacteria. *Bacteriol. Rev.* 39, 144−167.

[4]   Hoshino, T., Xiao, N., Yajima, Y. and Tkachenko, O.B. (2013). Fungi in cryosphere: Their adaptation to environments. In: Yumoto, I. editor. *Cold-adapted microorganisms.* Portland: Caister Academic Press.

[5]   Hoshino, T. and Matsumoto, N. (2012). Cryophilic fungi to denote fungi in the cryosphere. *Fungal Biol. Rev.*, 26, 102−105.

[6]   Hibbett, D.S., Binder, M., Bischoff, J.F., Blackwell, M., Cannon, P., Eriksson, O.E., Huhndorf, S., James, T., Kirk, P.M., Lücking, R., Thorsten Lumbsch, H., Lutzoni, F., Matheny, P.B., McLaughlin, D.J., Powell, M.J., Redhead, S., Schoch, C.L., Spatafora, J.W., Stalpers, J.A., Vigalys, R., Aime, M.C., Aptroot, A., Bauer, R., Begerow, D., Benny, G.L., Castlebury, L.A., Crous, P.W., Dai, Y.-C., Gams, W., Geiser, D.M., Griffith, G.W., Gueidan, C., Hawksworth, D.L., Hestmark, G., Hosaka, K., Humber, R.A., Hyde, K.D., Ironside, J.E., Kõljalg, U., Kurtzman, C.P., Larsson, K.-H., Lichtwardt, R., Longcore, J., Miądlikowska, J., Miller, A., Moncalvo, J.-M., Monzley-Standridge, S., Oberwinkler, F., Parmasto, E., Reeb, V., Rogers, J.D., Roux, C., Ryvarden, L., Sampaio, E., Schüßler, A., Sugiyama, J., Thorn, R.G., Tibell, L., Untereiner, W.A., Walker, C., Wang, Z., Weir, A., Weiss, M., White, M.M., Winka, K., Yao, Y.-J. and Zhang, N. (2007). A higher-level phylogenetic classification of the *Fungi. Mycol. Res.*, 111, 509–547.

[7]   Nedbalová, L., Kociánová, M. and Lukavský, J. (2008). Ecology of snow algae in the Giant Mts. *Opera Corcontica* 45, 59–68.

[8]   Kol, E. (1968). *Kryobiologie. Biologie und Limnologie des Schnees und Elises. I. Kryovegetation.* Stuttgart: E. Schweizerbart'sche Verlagebuchhandlung.

[9]   Kol, E. (1974). Trachiscia (Chlorophyta) red snow from Swedish Lapland. *Ann. Hist-Nat. Mus. Nat. Hung.* 66, 59–63.

[10] Kol, E. (1939). Zur Schneevegetation Patagoniens. *Ark. Bot. (Stockholm)*, 29, 1–4.

[11] Kol, E. (1942). The snow and ice algae of Alaska. *Smithsonian Misc. Collect.* 101, 1–36.

[12] Stein, J.R. and Amundsen, C.C. (1967). Studies on snow algae and fungi from the front range of Colorado. *Can. J. Bot.*, 45. 2033–2045.

[13] Kobayashi, Y. and Ôkubo, M. (1954). Studies on the aquatic fungi of the Ozegahara moor. Scientific researches of the Ozegahara moor. Editor. *Scientific Researches of the Ozegahara Moor -1954-.* Tokyo: JST; pp. 561–575.

[14] Kobayashi, Y. and Konno, K. (1986). *Icones of the Japanese water moulds with precise explantion.* Tokyo; Kobayashi, Y. and Konno, K.

[15] Hoham, R.W. and Duval, B. (2001). Microbial ecology of snow and freshwater ice with emphasis on snow algae. In: Jones, H.G., Pomeroy, J.W., Walker, D.A. and Hoham, R.W., editors. *Snow ecology. An interdisplinary examination of snow −covered ecosystems.* Cambridge: Cambridge University Press; pp. 168–228.

[16] Freedman, K.R., Martin, A.P., Karki, D., Lynch, R.C., Mitter, M.S., Meyer, A.F., Longcore, J.E., Simmons, D.R. and Schmidt, S.K. (2009). Evidence that chytrids dominate fungal communities in high-elevation soils. *Proc. Natl. Acad. Sci. USA*, 106, 18315–18320.

[17] Schmidt, S.K., Naff, C.S. and Lynch, R.C. (2012). Fungal communities at the edge: Ecological lessons from high alpine fungi. *Fugal Ecol.*, 5, 443–452.

[18] Sparrow, F.K. Jr. (1960). *Aquatic Phycomycetes.* Ann Arbor: University of Michigan Press.

[19] Gleason, F.H., Carney, L.T., Lilje, O. and Glockling, S.L. (2012). Ecological potentials of species of *Rozella* (Cryptomycota). *Fungal Ecol.* 5, 651–656.

[20] Boyce, J.S. (1961). *Forest pathology.* New York: McGraw-Hill.

[21] Bauer, H. and Schwaninger, C. (2007). Phytopathogens at the Alpine timberline. In: Wieser, G. and Tausz, M., editors. *Trees at their upper limit. Treelife limitation at the Alpine timberline*. Berlin: Springer ; pp. 163−170.

[22] Reid, J. and Cain, R.F. (1962). Studies on the organisms associated with "snow-blight" of conifers in North America. II. Some species of the genera *Phacidium, Lophophacidium, Sarcotrichila*, and *Hemiphacidium*. *Mycologia*, 54, 481−497.

[23] Roll-Hansen, F.R. (1989). Phacidium infestans. A literature review. *Eur. J. For. Path.*, 19, 237−250.

[24] Hoshino, T., Xiao, N. and Tkachenko, O.B. (2009). Cold adaptation in the phytopathogenic fungi causing snow molds. *Mycoscience*, 50, 26−38.

[25] Smerlis, E. (1968). Ascospore discharge of *Lophophacidium hyperboreum* and *Phacidium abietis*. *Bi-monthly Res. Note*, 24, 42.

[26] Kurkela, T. (1995). Short-term variation in ascospore release by *Phacidium infestans* on needles of *Pinus sylvestris*. *Eur. J. For. Path.*, 25, 274−281.

[27] Kurkela, T. (1996). Ascospore production period of *Phacidium infestans*, a snow blight fungus on *Pinus sylvestris*. *Scand. J. For. Res.*, 11, 60−67.

[28] Björkman, E. (1948). Studier över snöskyttesvampens snöskyttets bekämpande. *Meddel. Skogsforsk. Inst.* 37, 43−136.

[29] Lijia, A., Poteri, M., Petäistö, R.-L., Rikala, R., Kurkela, T. and Kasanen, R. (2010). Fungal dieases in forst nursearies in Finland. *Silva Fennica*, 44, 525−545.

[30] Petäistö, R.-L. and Laine, A. (1999). Effects of winter storage temperature and age of Scots pine seedlings on the occurrence of disease induced by *Gremmeniella abietina*. *Scand. J. For. Res.*, 14, 277−233.

[31] Yokota, S., Uozumi, T. and Matsuzaki, S. (1974). *Scleroderris* canker of Todo-fir in Hokkaido, northern Japan II. Physiological and pathological characteristics of the causal fungus. *Eur. J. For. Path.*, 4, 155−166.

[32] Akimoto, M. (1992). A new canker disease of *Cornus controversa* caused by *Microsphaeropsis* sp. (in Japnese). *Trans. Mtg. Hokkaido Br. Jpn. For. Soc.*, 40, 27−29.

[33] Hoham, R.W. and Mullet, J.E. (1977). The life history and ecology of the snow alga *Chloromonas cryophila* sp. nov. (Chlorophyta, Volvocales). *Phycologia*, 16, 53−68.

[34] Hoham, R.W. (1975). The life history and ecology of the snow alga *Chloromonas pinchinchae* (Chlorophyta, Volvocales), *Phycologia*, 14, 213−226.

[35] Smith, J.D., Jackson, N. and Woolhouse, A.R. (1989). *Fungal diseases of amenity turf grasses*. London: E. and F.N. Spon.

[36] Matsumoto, N. and Hoshino, T. (2009). Fungi in snow environments: Psychrophilic molds−A groups of pathogens affecting plants under snow. In: Misra, J.K. and Deshmukh, S.K., editors. *Fungi from different environments*. Enfield, Science Publishers: pp. 169−188.

[37] Årsvoll, K. (1975). Fungi causing winter damage on cultivated grasses in Norway. *Meld. Norg. Landbrukshøgsk.* 54(9), 1−49.

[38] Tkachenko, O.B. (2013). Snow mold fungi in Russia. In: Imai, R., Yoshida, M. and Matsumoto, N., editors. *Plant and Microbe Adaptations to Cold in a Changing World: Proceedings of the Plant and Microbe Adaptation to Cold Conference, 2012*. New York: Springer; in press.

[39] Terui, M. (1941). *Typhula japonica* n. sp. isolated from decayed leaves of the rape plant. *Trans. Sapporo Nat. Hist. Soc.*, 17, 40−49.

[40] Ito, K. (1975). *Pathology of forest trees III* (in Japanese). Tokyo: Nòrin Shuppan.

[41] Hoshino, T., Tkachenko, O.B., Kiriaki, M., Yumoto, I., Matsumoto, N. (2004). Winter damage caused by *Typhula ishikariensis* biological species I on conifer seedlings and hop roots collected in the Volga-Ural regions of Russia. *Can. J. Plant Pathol.* 26, 391–396.

[42] Woodbridge, B., Coley-Smith, J.R. and Reid, D.A. (1989). A new species of *Cylindrobasidium* parasitic on sclerotia of *Typhula incaranata*. *Trans. Br. Mycol. Soc.*, 91, 166–169.

[43] Kohn, L.M. and Nagasawa, E. (1984). The genus Scleromitula (Sclerotiniaceae), Episclerotium gen. nov. (Leotiaceae) and allied stipitate-capitate species with reduced ectal excipula. *Trans. Mycol. Soc. Jpn.*, 25, 127–148.

[44] Yajima, Y., Inaba, S., Degawa, Y., Hoshino, T. and Kondo, N. (2012). Ultrastructure of a cyst-like body in fruiting bodies of a snowbank myxomycete (plasmodial slime molds). *Plant and Microbe Adaptations to Cold 2012. Toward risk assessment and management of sustainable agriculture in the cool and cold regions.* pp. 89.

[45] Jones, M.D., Rhichards, T.A., Hawksworth, D.L. and Bass, D. (2011). Validation and justification of the phylum name *Cryptomycota* phyl. nov. *IMA Fungus*, 2, 173–175.

[46] Hoshino, T., Xiao, N., Yajima, Y., Kida, K., Tokura, K., Murakami, R., Tojo, M. and Matsumoto, N. (2013). Ecological strategies of snow molds to tolerate freezing stress. In: Imai, R., Yoshida, M. and Matsumoto, N., editors. *Plant and Microbe Adaptations to Cold in a Changing World: Proceedings of the Plant and Microbe Adaptation to Cold Conference, 2012.* New York: Springer; in press.

[47] Kusunoki, M. and Ichitani, T. (1982). Preparation of mycelium-free oospores of *Pythium butleri* by a freezing method. *Ann. Pytopath. Soc. Jpn.* 48, 695–698.

[48] Takamatsu, S. (1989). Snow molds in winter wheat: studies on occurrence of *Pythium* snow rot (in Japanese with English summary). *Spec. Bull. Fukui Agric. Exp. Stn.* 9, 1–135.

[49] Hoshino, T., Tojo, M., Kanda, H., Herrero, M.L., Tronsmo, A.M., Kiriaki, M., Yokota, Y. and Yumoto, I. (2002). Chilling resistance of isolates of *Pythium ultimum* var. *ultimum* from the Arctic and Temperate Zones. *Cryo-Lett.* 23, 151–156.

[50] Hoshino, T., Kiriaki, M., Ohgiya, S., Fujiwara, M., Kondo, H., Nihimiya, Y., Yumoto, I. and Tsuda, S. (2003). Antifreeze proteins from snow molds. *Can. J. Bot.* 81, 1175–1181.

[51] Hoshino, T., Terami, F., Tkachenko, O.B., Tojo, M. and Matsumoto, N. (2010). Mycelial growth of the snow mold fungus, *Sclerotinia borealis* improved at low water potentials: an adaptation to frozen environment. *Mycoscience* 51, 98–102.

[52] Wolf, F.A. and Wolf, F.T. (1947). *The Fungi Volume II.* New York: John Wiley and Sons.

[53] Kurkela, T. (1969). Antagonism of healthy and diseased ericaceous plants to snow blight on scot pine. *Acta For. Fenn.*, 101, 1–7.

[54] Matsumoto, N. and Tajimi, A. (1988). Life-history strategy in *Typhula incarnata* and *T. ishikariensis* biotypes A, B, and C as determined by sclerotium production. *Can. J. Bot.*, 66, 2485–2590.

[55] Hsiang, T., Matsumoto, N. and Millett, S. (1999). Biology and management of Typhula snow molds of turfgrass. *Plant Dis.* 83, 788–798.

[56] Satô, K. Pre-emergence damping-off coniferous seedlings caused by the pathogenic fungi of snow blight at low temperature (1) (in Japanese with English summary). *J. Jpn. For. Soc.*, 46, 171–177.

[57] McBeath, J.H. (1988). Sclerotinia myceliogenic germination and pathogenicity of *Sclerotinia borealis*. *5th Int. Cong. Plant Path., Kyoto*, pp. 201.

[58] Bruehl, G.W., Srague, R., Fischer, W.B., Nagamitsu, M., Nelson, W.L. and Vogel, O.A. (1966). Snow mold of winter wheat in Washington. *Wash. Agric. Stn. Bull.* 677, 1–21.

[59] Ono, K. (194). Studies on "Ezo-raigan" diseas, sclerotium germination-loss, of Todo-fir seeds (in Japanese with English abstract). *Bull. Gov. For. Exp. Stn.*, 268, 49–80.

[60] Coley-Smith, J.R. and Cooke, R.C. (1971). Survival and germination of fungal sclerotia. *Ann. Rev. Phytopathol.*, 9, 65–92.

[61] Tkachenko, O.B. (1997). Particularities of low-temperature basidiomycete *Typhula ishikariensis* in Russia. In: *Proceedings of International Workshop on Plant-Microbe Interactions at Low Temperature Under Snow.* Sapporo: Hokkaido National Agricultural Experimental Station, pp. 77–87.

[62] Davidson, R.M.Jr. and Bruehl, G.W. (1972). Factors affecting the effectiveness of sclerotia of *Typhula idahoensis* as inoculum. *Phytopaphology*, 62, 1040–1045.

[63] Tkachenko, O.B. (1995). Adaptation of the fungus *Typhula ishikariensis* Imai to the soil inhabitance (in Russian with English summary). *Mikol. Fitol.*, 29, 14–19.

[64] Tojo M, van West P, Hoshino T, Kida K, Fujii H, Hakoda C, Kawaguchi Y, Mühlhauser HA, van den Berg AH, Küpper FC, Herrero ML, Klemsdal SS, Tronsmo AM, Kanda H (2012) *Pythium polare*, a new heterothallic Oomycete causing grown discoloration of *Sanionia uncinata* in the Arctic and Antarctic. *Fugal Biology* 116:756–768.

[65] Tojo, M. and Newsham, K.K. (2012). Snow moulds in polar environments. *Fugal Ecol.*, 5, 395–402.

[66] Bridge, P.D., Newsham, K.K. and Denton, G.J. (2008). Snow mould caused by a *Pythium* sp.: a potential vascular plant pathogen in the maritime Antarctic. *Plant Pathol.*, 57, 1066–1072.

[67] Lebeau, J.B. and Longston, C.E. (1958). Snow mold of forage crops in Alaska and Yukon. *Phytopathology*, 48, 148–150.

[68] Hoshino, T., Saito, I., Yumoto, I. and Tronsmo, A.M. (2006). New findings of snow mold fungi from Greenland. *Medd. Grønland Biosci.*, 56, 89–94.

[69] Kristinsson, H. and Guðleifsson, B.E. (1976). The activity of low temperature fungi under the snow cover in Iceland. *Acta Bot. Isl.*, 4, 44–57.

[70] Jamalainen, E.A. (1949). Overwintering of *Gramineae* plants and parasitic fungi. I. *Sclerotinia borealis* Bubák and Vleugel. *J. Sci. Agric. Soc. Finl.*, 21, 125–142.

[71] Jamalainen, E.A. (1957). Overwintering of *Gramineae* plants and parasitic fungi. II. On the *Typhula* sp. fungi in Finland. *J. Sci. Agric. Soc. Finl.*, 29, 75–81.

[72] Ekstrand, H. (1955). Höstsädens och vallgräsens överwintering. *Statens Växtskyddsanstalt Meddelande*, 67, 1–125.

[73] Khokhryakova, T.M. (1983). Typhula blight and sclerotinia rot affection of grasses on the north and the north-west of the nonchernozem zone of the RSFSR. (in Russian, with English abstract). *Bull. Appl. Bot. Genet. Plant Breed.*, 82, 45–51.

[74]   Shiryaev, A.G. (2006). Clavarioid fungi of the Urals. III. Arctic zone (in Russian with English summary). *Mikol. Fitol.*, 40, 294−306.

[75]   Hoshino, T., Saito, I. and Tronsmo, A.M. (2003). Two snow mold fungi from Svalbard. *Lidia*, 6, 30−32.

[76]   Shirtaev, A.G. and Mukhin, V.A. (2010). Clavarioid-type fungi from Svalbard: Their spatial distribution in the European High Arctic. *North Am. Fungi*, 5, 67−84.

[77]   Gamundi, I.J. and Spinedi, H.A. (1987). Sclerotinia antarctica sp. nov., The teleomorph of the first fungus described Antarctica. *Mycotaxon*, 29, 81−89.

[78]   Yamazaki, Y., Tojo, M., Hoshino, T., Kida, K., Sakamoto, T., Ihara, H., Yumoto, I., Tronsmo, A.M. and Kanda, H. (2011). Characterization of *Trichoderma polysporum* from Spitsbergen, Svalbard archipelago, Norway, on species identity, infectivity to moss, and polygalacturonase activity. *Fungal Ecol.* 4, 15−21.

[79]   Tojo, M. and Nishitani, S. (2005). The effects of the smut fungus *Microbotryum bistotarum* on survival and growth of *Polygonum vivparum* in Svalbard. *Can. J. Bot.*, 83, 1513−1517.

[80]   Greenfield, L. (1983). Thermophilic fungi and actinomycetes from Mt. Erebus and fungus pathogenic to *Bryum antarcticum* at Cape Bird., *NZ. Antarctic Record 4*, 10-11.

[81]   Hawksworth, D.L. (1973). *Thyronectria antarctica* (Speg.) Seeler var. *hyperantarctica* D. Hawksw. var. nov. *Br. Antarc. Surv. Bull.*, 32, 51−53.

[82]   Longton, R.E. (1973). The occurrence of radial infection patterns in colonies of polar bryophytes. *Br. Antarc. Surv. Bull.*, 32, 41−49.

[83]   Fenton, J.H.C. (1983). Concentric fungal rings in Antarctic moss communities. *Tr. Br. Mycol. Soc.*, 80, 413−420.

[84]   Taylor, T. N., Galtier, J. and Axsmith, B. J. (1994). Fungi from the Lower Carboniferous of central France. *Rev. Palaeobot. Palynol.*, 83, 253−260.

[85]   Sakai, A. (1995). Shokubutsu no bunpu to kannkyō tekiō (in Japanese; Plant distribution and environmental adaptation). Tokyo: Asakura Publishing Co.

[86]   Matsumoto, N. (1997). Evolution and adaptation in snow mold fungi (in Japanese). Soil Microorganisms, 50, 13−19.

[87]   Hoshino, T. (2005). Ecophysiology of snow mold fungi. *Curr. Topic Plant Biol.*, 6, 27−36.

[88]   Ozerskaya, S., Kochkina, G., Ivanushkina, N. and Gilichinsky, D.A. (2009). Fungi in Permafrost. In: Margesin, R. editor. *Permafrost Soils, Soil Biology 16*. Berlin: Springer-Verlag, pp 85−95.

[89]   Stakhov, V.L., Gubin, S.V., Maksimovich, S.V., Rebrikov, D.V., Savilova, A.M., Kochkina, G.A., Ozerskaya, S.M., Ivanushkina, N.E. and Vorobyva, E.A. (2008). Microbial communities of ancient seeds derived from permanently frozen Pleistocene deposits. *Mikrobiologia*, 77, 348−355.

[90]   Matsumoto, N. (1992). Evolutionary ecology of the pathogenic species of *Typhula*. *Trans. Mycol. Soc. Jpn.*, 33, 269−285.

[91]   Matsumoto, N. (1994). Ecological adaptations of low temperature plant pathogenic fungi to diverse winter climates. *Can. J. Plant Pathol.*, 16, 237−240.

In: Advances in Medicine and Biology. Volume 69
Editor: Leon V. Berhardt
ISBN: 978-1-62808-088-9
© 2013 Nova Science Publishers, Inc.

Chapter VI

Commentary:
Molecular Basis of Hemibiotrophy in the Lentil Anthracnose Pathogen *Colletotrichum truncatum*

*Vijai Bhadauria and Sabine Banniza**
Crop Development Center, University of Saskatchewan, Saskatoon, Canada

Abstract

Hemibiotrophic fungal plant pathogens cause enormous economic damage to important food crops, such as cereals, legumes and oil seeds. These pathogens have two distinct *in planta* growth phases, an initial symptomless biotrophic and a subsequent destructive necrotrophic phase where the switch to necrotrophy is critical for disease development. Our recent studies indicate that pathogens likely secrete effector proteins to induce a hypersensitive cell death response triggered precisely before the switch to necrotrophy, and this cell death is critical for morphological and genetic differentiation of intracellularly proliferating secondary fungal hyphae. Toxins and hydrolyzing enzymes likely amplify cell death signals to accommodate the pathogen life-style. Here, we provide novel insight into the role of effectors in the hemibiotrophic parasitism of *Colletotrichum truncatum*, the causative agent of lentil anthracnose.

Based on the infection process and the mode of how fungal pathogens feed on their host plants, they can be classified into three main groups: biotrophs, necrotrophs and hemibiotrophs. Biotrophic pathogens like *Erysiphe cichoracearum* (causal agent of cucumber and *Arabidopsis* powdery mildew) inject their feeding structures (haustoria) into host plants

---

* Correspondence Author's Email address: sabine.banniza@usask.ca

and derive nutrients from living tissues to support their growth and reproduction on the host surface. This type of plant-fungal pathogen interaction follows the gene-for-gene hypothesis. The presence of matching pairs of resistance genes in the host plant and effector (avirulence) genes in the pathogen causes a rapid and localized hypersensitive cell death response (HR), which is sufficient to halt the ingress of the pathogen. The absence of or mutation in one or both partners (genes) causes compatibility, which is manifested by disease symptoms. Necrotrophic pathogens like *Sclerotinia sclerotiorum* (causal agent of multi-host white mould disease) overwhelm their host plants by secreting toxins and hydrolyzing enzymes (cell wall degrading enzymes and proteases), which allow them to subsist on dead or necrotised plant tissues. Some necrotrophs like *Pyrenophora tritici-repentis* produce host-selective toxins and induce symptoms in those genotypes of the host species that possess the matching toxin receptors. Hence, this type of plant - fungal pathogen interaction follows the reverse of the gene-for-gene hypothesis and is known as the toxin model. The presence of matching pair of toxin receptor gene(s) in the plant host and toxin gene in the pathogen cause compatibility, whereas the absence of or mutation in one or both partners leads to failure in disease development. The third group of fungal pathogens is known as hemibiotrophic pathogens, which include pathogens of high economic significance, such as *Colletotrichum* spp. (C. *truncatum*, *C. higginsianum* and *C. graminicola*), *Setosphaeria turcica*, *Leptosphaeria maculans*, *Mycosphaerella fijiensis* and *Magnaporthe oryzae*. These pathogens employ a sequential biotrophic and necrotrophic infection strategy to colonize their host plants [1].

Anthracnose caused by *Colletotrichum truncatum* (Schwein.) *Andrus and Moore* is one of the most devastating diseases of lentil (*Lens culinaris* Medik.) grown in western Canada. This fungal pathogen is a specialized hemibiotrophic pathogen that employs a two-stage infection strategy to colonize lentil plants. After penetration via appressoria, *C. truncatum* forms thick primary hyphae that are biotrophic in nature. The biotrophic phase and primary hyphae are entirely confined to the initially infected epidermal cells. No visible symptom is observed during the biotrophic phase. Water-soaked necrotic lesions become visible when the pathogen starts switching to the necrotrophic phase, which is associated with the differentiation of thin filamentous secondary hyphae emanating from the biotrophic primary hyphae. Therefore, the morphological and genetic switch to necrotrophy (biotrophy-necrotrophy switch, BNS) is critical in anthracnose development [2].

Despite being a decisive factor in the manifestation of diseases, to date only a handful of studies based on random insertional mutagenesis (RIM) have been published to address this important BNS. RIM is a powerful reverse genetics tool to dissect the biological functions of individual genes. Over a decade ago, Dufresne and colleagues [3] screened a RIM library of *C. lindemuthianum*, the causative agent of anthracnose on common bean (*Phaseolus vulgaris*) and identified a mutant H433 that elicited a hypersensitive cell death response on common bean leaves. Cytological analysis revealed a blockage of the switch to necrotrophy. Sequences flanking to the insertion site in the genome were retrieved by the plasmid rescue approach, which led to the identification of *CLTA1* (*Colletotrichum lindemuthianum transcriptional activator 1*) gene. The *CLTA1* encodes a transcription factor belonging to the zinc cluster (Zn[II]$_2$Cys$_6$) or GAL4 family. Targeted disruption of the *CLTA1* showed that this transcription factor is indispensable for the BNS. However, the mechanism by which the CLTA1 regulates the switch remained ambiguous. A relationship between nitrogen starvation and the BNS was eventually established as *C. lindemuthianum* requires CLNR1, an AREA and NIT2 (global fungal nitrogen regulators)-like protein for utilizing nitrogen sources.

Targeted deletion of the *CLNR1* gene impaired the BNS though mutants were similar to the wild-type up to the end of the biotrophic phase, suggesting that nitrogen starvation in the host plant acts as a cue to activate such BNS regulatory genes [4]. Restriction enzyme and *Agrobacterium tumefaciens*-mediated RIM libraries were constructed to identify pathogenicity genes from *C. graminicola* (causal agent of leaf blight and stalk rot of maize) and *C. higginsianum* (causal agent of anthracnose on cruciferous plants) [5, 6]. Two RIM mutants showed impairment in the initiation of the necrotrophic phase, but were indistinguishable from their respective wild-type strain until the end of the biotrophic phase. A plasmid rescue approach confirmed that the mutant from *C. graminicola* was disrupted in the *CPR1* locus, and the *C. higginsianum* mutant in a gene encoding importin-β2. *CPR1* encodes a putative eukaryotic microsomal signal peptidase, suggesting that the gene is required for secretion of hydrolyzing enzymes to support the BNS. However, unlike Δ*clta1* and Δ*clnr1*, *CPR1* is an essential gene as no viable transformant was obtained during an attempt to knock-out the gene. Whole genome sequencing followed by transcriptome profiling of *C. higginsianum* and *C. graminicola* provided a snapshot of genes potentially regulating different infection stages, such as expression of genes coding for effectors and secondary metabolism enzymes (SMEs) induced prior to fungal invasion and during the biotrophic phase, and hydrolyzing enzymes and transporters-encoding genes elevated at the switch to necrotrophy [7]. More recently, two other *Colletotrichum* spp. (*C. gloeosporiodes* and *C. orbiculare*) were sequenced and analyzed, highlighting fungal pathogenicity features. In both genomes, expansions of gene families were found that contained genes encoding small secreted proteins (putative effectors), SMEs, proteases and carbohydrate-degrading enzymes). By transcriptome analysis, the authors showed a hemibiotrophic phase shift of *C. orbiculare* during *Nicotiana tabacum* colonization [8].

Recently in an interesting study, a mitochondrial alternative oxidase (AOX) was identified in the witches' broom basidiomycete pathogen *Moniliophthora perniciosa* and shown to be indispensable for the transition from monokaryotic biotrophic hyphae to dikaryotic necrotrophic hyphae with clamp connections. The AOX catalyzes the reduction of O_2 to H_2O and provides an alternative respiratory route to the conserved cytochrome-dependent respiratory chain, which can be inhibited by nitric oxide generated during in host milieu to combat pathogen infection [9]. Research conducted to date, on elucidating the molecular mechanisms underlying the BNS suggested that hemibiotrophic phytopathogens secrete distinct classes of effector proteins that first hijack the plant basal and R-gene mediated defense to avert elicitation of a HR during the biotrophic phase, but then exploit the plant system to induce HR during the necrotrophic phase. A *suppressor of necrosis 1* (*SNE1*) effector gene was identified in the hemibiotrophic oomycete pathogen *Phytophthora infestans,* the causative agent of late blight of potato. *SNE1* was specifically expressed during the biotrophic phase and suppressed cell death induced by PiNPP1.1 (secreted during the necrotrophic phase), Avr-R protein interactions and PsojNIP (secreted during the switch to necrotrophy). This supports the hypothesis of sequential secretion of effector proteins with cell death-suppressing activity and cell death -inducing activity by hemibiotrophic pathogens to accommodate the life-style transition [10, 11]. Our recent research [12] provided further novel insight into the role of effectors in hemibiotrophic parasitism. We identified an effector protein named CtNUDIX (*C. truncatum* nucleoside diphosphate linked to moiety *X*) that *C. truncatum* secretes in lentil cells exclusively and precisely before the end of biotrophy to induce cell death. This cell death likely signals the switch to necrotrophy. CtNUDIX contains a nudix hydrolase domain (pfam00293). Nudix hydrolases are characterized by the presence of 23 amino acid nudix motif (GX$_5$EX$_7$REVXEEXGU, U = hydrophobic amino acid and X = any amino acid) and are known to hydrolyze a pyrophosphate bond of a nucleoside diphosphate linked to moiety X [13]. The moiety X can be a phosphate group (like nucleoside triphosphates and its oxidized form), a nucleoside with 2 to 6 phosphate groups (like diadenine polyphosphate), a nucleoside (which contains nicotinamide base in place of regular nitrogen base, such as NADH and NAD$^+$), a modified nucleoside, such as 7-methylguanosine (also known as mRNA cap), ribose sugar (like nucleotide sugar) or 4-phosphopantethenic acid (vitamin B$_5$) and β-mercaptoethylamine, such as Coenzyme A [13, 14].

Recently, the RXLR effector Avr3b identified from an oomycete pathogen *Phytophthora sojae*, the causal agent of soybean root rot disease was shown to have NUDIX hydrolase activity. The Av3b hydrolyzes NADH and ADP-ribose substrates to suppress host defense responses, such as accumulation of reactive oxygen species around infection sites [15]. NUDIX hydrolase can also hydrolyze non-nucleoside derivatives, such as inositol pyrophosphate (IP, also known as diphosphoinositol polyphosphate [PP-InsP$_n$]) [16, 17, 18]. IP6 and 7 take part in clathrin-mediated endocytosis by binding adapter proteins in which the plant plasma membrane invaginates and pinches off in form of vesicles containing extracellular molecules or non-self moleculaes, which are eventually degraded by hydrolytic enzymes present in lysosomes. These IPs are likely to participate in endocytosis via clathrin-coated pit assembly [19, 20]. CtNUDIX may hydrolyze IPs by breaking the pyrophosphate bond, which in turn affects endocytotic trafficking or cell membrane dynamics. This change in molecular dynamics could make the lentil cell membrane porous or permeable, which may allow the flooding of plant cells with non-native proteins that are subsequently recognized by the general surveillance system and induce cell death (a cue required for the switch to necrotrophy) (Figure 1). As evidence for this process, we showed that the chimeric CtNUDIX: eGFP proteins are initially localized in vesicle-like structures protruding towards the cytoplasm and cause HR in *N. tabacum* leaves. Overexpression of the CtNUDIX in *C. truncatum* and a second hemibiotrophic pathogen, *Magnaporthe oryzae* caused incompatibility with their host plants lentil and barley, respectively, by eliciting cell death during the biotrophic phase. CtNUDIX homologs are conserved among hemibiotrophic fungal pathogens, suggesting a common strategy exploited by these pathogens to colonize their host plants [2, 12, 21]. Therefore, NUDIX effectors could be an excellent target for the engineering resistance in host plants.

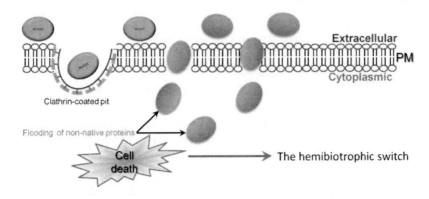

Figure 1. Putative model of CtNUDIX function. PM, plasma membrane.

Acknowledgments

This work was supported by Natural Sciences and Engineering Research Council of Canada and the Saskatchewan Pulse Growers Board.

References

[1] Glazebrook, J. (2005). Contrasting mechanisms of defense against biotrophic and necrotrophic pathogens. *Annual Review of Phytopathology*, 43, 205–227.

[2] Bhadauria, V. Banniza, S. Vandenberg, A. Selvaraj, G. and Wei, Y. (2011). EST mining identifies proteins secreted at the hemibiotrophic switch of the anthracnose pathogen *Colletotrichum truncatum*. BMC Genomics, 12, e327.

[3] Dufresne, M. Perfect, S. Pellier, A.L. Bailey, J.A. and Langin, T. (2000). A GAL4-like protein is involved in the switch between biotrophic and necrotrophic phases of the infection process of *Colletotrichum lindemuthianum* on common bean. *Plant Cell*, 12, 1579–1589.

[4] Pellier, A.L. Lauge, R., Veneault-Fourrey, C. and Langin, T. (2003). CLNR1, the AREA/NIT2-like global nitrogen regulator of the plant fungal pathogen *Colletotrichum lindemuthianum* is required for the infection cycle. *Molecular Microbiology*, 48, 635-655.

[5] Thon, M.R. Nuckles, E.M. Takach, J.E. and Vaillancourt, L.J. (2002). *CPR1*: A gene encoding a putative signal peptidase that functions in pathogenicity of *Colletotrichum graminicola* to maize. *Molecular Plant-Microbe Interactions*, 15, 120-128.

[6] Huser, A. Takahara, H. Schmalenbach, W. and O'Connell, R. (2009). Discovery of pathogenicity genes in the crucifer anthracnose fungus *Colletotrichum higginsianum*, using random insertional mutagenesis. *Molecular Plant-Microbe Interactions*, 22, 143-156.

[7] O'Connell, R.J. Thon, M.R. Hacquard, S. Amyotte, S.G. Kleemann, J. Torres, M.F. Damm, U. Buiate, E.A. Epstein, L. Alkan, N. Altmüller, J. Alvarado-Balderrama, L., Bauser, C.A., Becker, C., Birren, B.W., Chen, Z. Choi, J. Crouch, J.A. Duvick, J.P. Farman, M.A. Gan, P., Heiman, D. Henrissat, B. Howard, R.J. Kabbage, M. Koch, C. Kracher, B. Kubo, Y., Law, A.D. Lebrun, M. Lee, Y. Miyara, I. Moore, N. Neumann, U. Nordström, K. Panaccione, D.G. Panstruga, R. Place,M. Proctor, R.H. Prusky, D. Rech, G. Reinhardt, R. Rollins, J.A. Rounsley, S. Schardl, C.L. Schwartz, D.C. Shenoy, N. Shirasu, K. Sikhakolli, U.R. Stüber, K. Sukno, S.A. Sweigard, J.A. Takano, Y. Takahara, H. Trail, F. van der Does, H.C. Voll, L.M. Will, I. Young, S. Zeng, Q. Zhang, J. Zhou, S. Dickman, M.B. Schulze-Lefert, P. van Themaat, E.V.L, Ma, L. and Vaillancourt, L.J. (2012). Lifestyle transitions in plant pathogenic *Colletotrichum* fungi deciphered by genome and transcriptome analyses. *Nature Genetics*, 44(9), 1060-1065.

[8] Gan, P. Ikeda, K. Irieda, H. Narusaka, M. O'Connell, R.J. Narusaka, Y. Takano, Y. Kubo, Y. and Shirasu, K. (2013). Comparative genomics and transcriptomics analyses reveal the hemibiotrophic stage shift of *Colletotrichum* fungi. *New Phytologist*, 197(4), 1236-1249.

[9]   Thomazella, D.P.T. Teixeira, P.P.L. Oliveira, H.C. Saviani, E.E. Rincones, J.Toni, I.M. Reis, O. Garcia, O. Meinhardt, L.W. Salgado, I. and Pereira, G.A.G. (2012). The hemibiotrophic cacao pathogen *Moniliophthora perniciosa* depends on a mitochondrial alternative oxidase for biotrophic development. *New Phytologist*, 194, 1025–1034.

[10]   Kelley, B.S. Lee, S.J. Damasceno, C.M. Chakravarthy, S. Kim, B.D. Martin, G.B. and Rose, J.K. (2010). A secreted effector protein (SNE1) from *Phytophthora infestans* is a broadly acting suppressor of programmed cell death. *Plant Journal*, 62, 357–366.

[11]   Lee, S.J. and Rose, J.K.C. (2010). Mediation of the transition from biotrophy to necrotrophy in hemibiotrophic plant pathogens by secreted effector proteins. *Plant Signaling and Behavior*, 5, 769-772.

[12]   Bhadauria, V. Banniza, S. Vandenberg, A. Selvaraj, G. and Wei, Y. (2013). Overexpression of a novel biotrophy-specific *Colletotrichum truncatum* effector CtNUDIX in hemibiotrophic fungal phytopathogens causes incompatibility with their host plants. *Eukaryotic Cell*, 12(1), 2-11.

[13]   Mildvan, A.S. Xia, Z. Azurmendi, H.F. Saraswat, V. Legler, P.M. Massiah, M.A. Gabelli, S.B. Bianchet, M.A. Kang, L.W. and Amzel, L.M. (2005). Structures and mechanisms of Nudix hydrolases. *Achieves of Biochemistry and Biophysics*, 433, 129–143.

[14]   Bessman, M.J. Frick, D.N. and O'Handley, S.F. (1996). The MutT proteins or "Nudix" hydrolases, a family of versatile, widely distributed, "housecleaning" enzymes. *Journal of Biological Chemistry*, 271, 25059–25062.

[15]   Dong, S. Yin, W., Kong, G. Yang, X. Qutob, D. Chen, Q. Kale, S.D. Sui, Y. Zhang, Z. Dou, D. Zheng, X. Gijzen, M. Tyler, B.M. and Wang, Y. (2011). *Phytophthora sojae* avirulence effector Avr3b is a secreted NADH and ADP-ribose pyrophosphorylase that modulates plant immunity. *PLOS Pathogens* 7(11), e1002353.

[16]   Safrany, S.T. Caffrey, J.J. Yang, X. Bembenek, M.E. Moyer, M.B. Burkhart, W.A. and Shears, S.B. (1998). A novel context for the 'MutT' module, a guardian of cell integrity, in a diphosphoinositol polyphosphate phosphohydrolase. *EMBO Journal*, 17, 6599–6607.

[17]   Safrany, S.T. Ingram, S.W. Cartwright, J.L. Falck, J.R. McLennan, A.G. Barnes, L.D. and Shears, S.B. (1999). The diadenosine hexaphosphate hydrolases from *Schizosaccharomyces pombe* and *Saccharomyces cerevisiae* are homologs of the human diphosphoinositol polyphosphate phosphohydrolase. Overlapping substrate specificities in a MutT-type protein. *Journal of Biological Chemistry*, 274, 21735-21740.

[18]   Gabelli, S.B. Bianchet, M.A. Xu, W. Dunn, C.A. Niu, Z.D. Amzel, L.M. and Bessman, M.J. (2007). Structure and function of the *E. coli* dihydroneopterin triphosphates pyrophosphatase: a Nudix enzyme involved in folate biosynthesis. *Structure*, 15, 1014-1022.

[19]   Saiardi, A., Resnick, A.C., Snowman, A.M., Wendland, B. and Snyder, S.H. (2005). Inositol pyrophosphates regulate cell death and telomere length through phosphoinositide 3-kinase-related protein kinases. *PNAS*, 102(6), 1911-1914.

[20] Saiardi, A. Sciambi, C. McCaffery, J.M. Wendland, B. and Snyder, S.H. (2002). Inositol pyrophosphates regulate endocytotic trafficking. *PNAS*, 99(2), 14206-14211.

[21] Bhadauria, V. Banniza, S. Vandenberg, A. Selvaraj, G. and Wei, Y. (2011). Cataloging proteins putatively secreted during the biotrophy-necrotrophy transition of the anthracnose pathogen *Colletotrichum truncatum*. *Plant Signaling and Behavior,* 6(10), 1457–1459.

In: Advances in Medicine and Biology. Volume 69   ISBN: 978-1-62808-088-9
Editor: Leon V. Berhardt   © 2013 Nova Science Publishers, Inc.

Chapter VII

Detection of Gaze Atypical Pattern: A Systematic Review of Eye Tracking in the Autistic Spectrum Disorders

*Nuria Aresti Bartolomé, Begoña García Zapirain**
DeustoTech-Life Unit DeustoTech Institute of Technology
University of Deusto, Bilbao, Spain

Abstract

This chapter provides a review on the evolution of the Eye Tracking technology and the use of this technology in the detection of atypical patterns in people with autistic spectrum disorder (ASD). ASDs constitute one of the most serious mental diseases in the chilhood due to the complexity of its detection, diagnosis and treatment, despite the fact that its prevalence is lower than in other chilhood pathologies. For some decades now, the examination of the eye pattern in this collective has begun, due to the fact that they present an alteration in the use of multiple non-verbal behaviours, such as the eye contact. The studies conducted so far have been guided by two types of tests: videos with social /non-social scenes, or with static images. It has been proven the differences between the control groups and the people affected by ASD, and more precisely in those dynamic stimuli including social scenes, in which, the fixing in the eye contours diminishes, thus increasing in the regions or the body or other objects, being this a predictive element of the social response of these people. This chapter discusses the tendencies and results of the use of the Eye Tracking technology carried out to date within the field of the autistic spectrum disorder.

Keywords: Eye Tracking, Autistic Spectrum Disorders, gaze pattern, static images, videos

---

*E-mail address: {nuria.aresti,mbgarciazapi}@deusto.es

1. Introduction

Autistic Spectrum Disorders (ASD) constitute one of the most serious mental pathologies in chilhood, and this is due precisely to the difficulty of its detection, diagnosis and treatment [1] in spite of its prevalence being lower than other chilhood pathologies.

ASD or pervasive developmental disorders (PDD) are neuropsichiatric problems, which arc revealed before three years of age and affect to the cognitive, social and communication areas, accompanied by stereotyped behaviours [2] [3].

The term "autism" was first mentioned in 1912, in the "Dementia Praecox or the Group Schizophrenia" publication, conducted by the Swiss neuropsychiatrist Eugene Bleuler in the "American Journal of Insanity". The term "autism" comes from the Greek word "autos" , which means "Itself". Bleuler employed the term to define the active withdrawal the schizophrenic patients used to avoid the social relationships by means of the isolation towards the realm of fantasy [4], [5].

In En 1943, the Austrian Physician Leo Kanner described 11 children presenting a developmental disorder, which was defined as "autistic contact disorder" In thas studey, a series of features presented by the subjects were determined. [6].

- Difficulty with reciprocal social interactions, with extreme loneliness.

- Severe language and communication alterations.

- Obsesive enphasis in the invariance.

A year later, in 1944, the Austrian physician Hans Asperger, in a study conducted with 4 children between the ages of 6 and 11, defined a disorder similar to the one carried out by Kanner. Those children showed as a main feature the disability in the social interaction, but, unlike the autism presented by Kanner, those subjects did not present a significant delay, neither in cognitive development, nor in language acquisition. Hans Asperger defined it as "Chilhood autistic Psychopathy" [7].

In 1981, Lorna Wing presented a study reviewing Hans Asperger's work, by means of 34 cases in which a series of features similar to those explained by Asperger were described [8]. In this particular case, Lorna Wing suggested the "Asperger's Syndrome" to define the features of the cases object of study. Wing determined a dimensional diagnostic model, and proposed the hypothesis of the "Continuous autistic" (1988) with the aim of explaining the different degrees of affections in the nuclear deficits within this collective (Wing's Triad) [9]:

- Social relation disorder.

- Communication disorder, including language comprehension and expression.

- Lack of mental flexibility, which shapes a restricted number of conducts, and a limitation in the activities requiring certain degree of imagination.

In the light of these studies, the term Autistic Spectrum Disorder (ASD) is included. This ASD term adopts a dimensional concept of "continuous" (Not a category), thus existing other disorders that share some of the features included in the Wing's triad, and, additionally, there exist different degrees within the autistic spectrum depending on the lower, medium or higher cognoscitive level, and depending also on its greater or lesser symptomatology [9].

There exist two main ranking systems accepted and valued worldwide, in which the descriptions of the disorders, syndromes.. are based on symptomatological and behavioural aspects [10].

- Diagnostic and Statistical manual of mental disorders (DSM) . This manual was created by the American psychiatry association (APA) in 1952, and it is the most used system for the international quality research. Diverse versions of the DSM have been made, being the last published version the DSM-IV-TR. Therefore, in May 2013 there is another version to be published : DSM-V.

- Classification of mental disorders (CIE) Created by the World Health Organization (WHO). The CIE is used at European level.

In the DSM-IV-TR, the autism is shown as a pervasive developmental disorder, and it is divided into five subgroups: Asperger's syndrome, Non-specified pervasive disorder, Rett's syndrome, autistic disorder and Chilhood Disintegrative disorder. But, as far as these studies carried out is concerned, the limit among these developmental disorders is not clear enough, specially the difference between the Asperger's syndrome and the high functioning autism, since more similarities rather thant differences between them were found [11] , [12], [9]. Some authors maintain that the cases included in the PDD in the DSM-IV-R are imprecise, up to and including children with other type of disorders, such as attention deficit disorder and hyperactivity [2]. Due to these reasons, the new publication to be programmed in 2013 will entail a change in the group of PDD. This PDD concept will disappear giving rise to the "Autistic spectrum Disorder (ASD)". This concept was used after the studies conducted by Wing. The ASD serves to collect all the disorders sharing the deficits of the autism, but from a continuum or dimension [9]which are associated with a wide variety of features, symptoms, etymological factors [13].

The first published draft designs of the **DSM-V** establishes that the new ASD nomenclature includes the autistic disorder (autism), the Asperger's disorder, the Chilhood Disintegrative disorder and the non-specified pervasive developmental disorder [14].

The DSM-V includes another change with respect to the DSM-IV-TR related to the affectation domains. Up to the moment, with the DSM-IV-TR, the PDD affected to the social interaction, language, and symbolic or imaginative game [15], Notwithstanding, in the DSM-V the affectation domains will be reduced to two [16]:

- Social and Communication deficits: Deficits in communication and social behaviour are inseparable, and they can be considered in a more precise way as a unique set of symptoms with environmental and contextual specificities

- Fixed interests and repetitive behaviour

The language is removed, since it is determined that the delays in the language are not unique and universal in ASD, and, more precisely, it can be considered as a factor that influences in the clinical symptoms of ASD, instead of defining the diagnosis, as it has been made thus far.

One of the features that stablish either the CIE and the DSM, both in the DSM-IV-TR version and the DSM-V version, is that people with the autistic spectrum disorder present an alteration in the eye contact. From the year 2000 onwards, a series of studies and research works started, in order to be able to evaluate objectively the atypical contact within the affected persons. To do so, the technology called **eye Tracking** was employed, which allows the obtention of a register of the eye-monitoring.

This chapter presents the historical evolution of the eye tracking technology, as well as the research works and uses of this tenchology within the field of the ASD.

2. Historical Evolution

The Eye Tracking concept makes reference to a set of technologies that allow the monitoring and registering the way a person stares at a determined scene or image, that is to say, in which areas the attention is focused, during how long and what order follows in the visual exploration [17].

The study of the movement of the eyes has been performed for more than 100 years. The preliminary studies about eye movement were carried out by direct observation or by introspection, with the assistance of mirrors, telescopes, [18]. Louis Emile Javal in 1879 was the first one who studied the eye movement while reading, thus identifying rapid movements or "saccades" and short stops while reading instead of undertaking a smooth sweeping.

Edmud Delabarre, analysed the eye movement employing a hat connected to the eyes through a cable. This cable, in turn, is linked to a lever that drew the motion in a kymograph (A device that registers the signals coing from the movement of an organ or optical device) [18]. In 1900, Edmunf Huey presented an invasive system using a sort of contact lens with a hole, connected to an aluminium pointer that moved in response to the eye movement.

The methods used by Delabarre and Huey involved the contact of a device directly to the cornea, until 1991, when Dodge and Cline invented the first non-invasive system, by means of the use of beam-lines emission. The system consisted on the emission of beam-lines to the eyes, and its reflect was recorded through photography. This was the first research work conducted concerning eye movement, using the reflection of the cornea. This method is the one used by the experts, even nowadays.

During the 1920s, in the laboratories of Chicago and Standford, the first eye movement registers begun, in three dimensions, by capturing simultaneously two images of the eye. Later on, the decomposition of the light beam reflection in an eye in its horizontal and vertical components was overcome. Buswell in 1935 used this decomposition of the beam reflection to measure the analysis routes of a subject while observing an image [19] [18].

Up to 1970 the methods measured the eye movement with respect to the head, thus being essential the use of external device to maintain the users' head motionless. Nevertheless, in this decade two optical features of the eyes started to be used; This is why the fixing systems were abandoned.

Consequently, the eye tracking systems count with a main feature: Its invasive or non invasive nature [20],being the latter the one most accepted by the users due to its convenience. Similarly, eye tracking systems can be classified by means of the methodology used for the eye movement measurements: ElectroOculoGram(EOG),video-oculography (VOG), photo oculography (POG) or Contact lens- based systems.

The clustering of such pathologies, described on the basis of its invasive and non invasive nature are going to be shown hereafter.

a) **Non invasive systems**. These systems are those in which there is no contact between the device and the user. In the eye-tracking systems, it is undertaken through infrared light, which is reflected in the users' eyes and it is captured by a camera or any optical sensor.

 – Photo-oculography (POG) and Video-oculography (VOG) The basic elements of an eye-tracking elements based on video oculography are the light sources and the image acquisition system employed. In this system a videocamara observes the user's eye and an image processing software will be given the task of analysing the video image of the eye and determines, in real time, the coordinates of the place on the screen where the eye points to [21]. Those systems use the the reflection of the pupil /cornea centre to determine the direction of the eye. To do so, a low-power infrared light is emitted from a LED, located in the middle of the lens of the camera illuminating the eye. The pupil centre, the contour of the iris, and the reflections of the cornea are analysed, thus endeavouring to establish a relation between such reflections and the place where the gaze is fixed; That is to say, it stares at the eye orientation in the "point of regard" space (PoR) [18].

b) **Invasive systems** These systems are the ones requiring the contact of the system with the subject. Those systems, though more reliable, tend to be inconvenient for the users/subjects, thus being the non-invasive systems better accepted.

 – Systems based on contact lenses. These systems are the ones more precise, due to the fact that the device is in direct contact and adjusted to the eye. Special lenses systems are employed, composed by two individual spherical surfaces that are adjusted over the cornea and the sclera. The contact lens and the material associated to such lens should not be of such volume and size that may interfere with eye movements.

c) **Electrical potentials** This method uses the electrical potential measured with electrodes placed around the eyes to detect the movement. The ayes are the origin of a constant electrical potential field, which can also be detected in total darkness, even though the eyes are closed.

 – ElectroOculoGram (EOG). The ElectroOculoGram (EOG) registers the voltage variations occurring with the angular movement of the eye. The obtention of the EOG placing a system of perbiocular silver electrodes-silver chloride and a bioelectric conduction gel as an electrolite in the electrode interface-skin. With this electrode configuration, a series of signals in independent derivations either vertical or horizontal can be achieved, also combining them to obtain almost every type of eye movement [22].

As stated above, the non-invasive movements are the most accepted by the users. More-over, they can be grouped in two types of systems:

- Systems placed over the user's head

- Remote systems

The former ones are appropriate to carry out a register of rapid head movements or, in systems in which the user requires freedom of movements.

Notwithstanding, these systems are not advisable in systems in which a continuous gaze during a long span of time is needed, as it can occur in the cursor control for people with motor disability, or in applications involving children. For these applications, the second group, named remote systems are more adequate, since they are non-invasive children and they are not in contact with the users. These systems are commonly located or integrated in the monitors, and they register the eye movement from the distance [23].

2.1. EyeTracker commercial systems

The market offers different companies that develop eye tracking systems, which are vali-dated by different studies. A selection of the most commonly used systems is carried out thereupon:

- EYELINKII

  EyeLink II is developed by the SR Research Complete Eye Tracking Solutions com-pany. It consists of three minicameras placed in a padded headband over the head. The two eye cameras allow the precise tracking of the eyes.

- FACELAB5

  FaceLab5 is created by "seeingmachines" and it generates data from the following captured parameters: Eye movement, head position and rotation, lid-opening, lip and eyebrow movement, and pupil size.

- S2 EYE TRACKER

  S2 Eye tracker allows to capture in real time the place the user is staring at. Some of the features of this system are: Precise, easy to use, flexible, portable, non invasive.

- Tobii TX300

  Tobii TX300 is a new remote eye tracker, with an intermediate sampling rate, which does not require the user to maintain the head static or in a chin strap. Its sampling rate of 300Hz, its high precision, its accuracy in the measurements and its great head movement compensation broaden the spectrum of research fields possible for the analysis of oculomotor functions and human behaviour.

- Tobii X1 light

  This system, is a more economic alternative than Tobii TX300, but it shares the main features, such as: The precision and accuracy, in the whole monitoring space (not only in the middle), the IR variable illumination pattern and double captation camera, which results in high fidelity and data gathering accuracy along the whole screen range, high robustness to the illumination changes, non intrusive, and there is no need the user to employ a chin strap, and a high robustness to the head movements of the user during the test.

3. Eye Tracking Use Tendencies

The eye tracking technology can be used for different purposes. At one end, it acts as a tool for the objective evaluation of interfaces [17].In the literature there exist multiple references to different studies conducted to check the usability of the aplications using eye tracking technologies, testing the design of the icons, the graphic representations, tables, the readability in texts, etc [23] [24], the search and information recovery interfaces [25],the digital media [26] and the on-line advertising impact have been also studied.

Another possible use is to employ it as an input or interaction device, in PCs, or in the interaction with videogames. This way, new experiences are created for the users, thus facilitating the game to people with reduced mobility, since the eye movement is employed as game control systems, that is to say, the act as though they are the mouse, or classic joystick [18].

4. Eye Tracking Tendencies and Research in ASD Collectives

The use of the Eye Tracking technology is specially oriented towards the detection of autistic features in people. To do so, this technology is also employed to obtain atypical patterns together with the fixation and interests of these people.

The results of the studies conducted in the detection and classification of ASD, as well as the gaze patterns obtained with the EyeTracking technology will be described thereupon.

4.1. ASD Detection

The Eye Tracking technology has been used in order to obtain objective indicators of a possible early detection of ASD. Within this field, there exist two tracks: Those indicating that the results obtained with this technology can be biomedical indicators of a possible case of ASD. The other track establishes that there is no sufficient difference between the control group and the group with ASD.

To be able to carry out these studies, different techniques or tests assessed with the Eye Tracking technology were employed.

- Still Face" technique

  LaThe "Still Face" technique consists on the evaluation of the child reaction to different expressions of their mother. To do so, the mother goes through different stages. In the first one the mother should interact with the child in a normal way, then, the child should be stared at without showing any type of expression and without reacting to the child's inquiries, and, finally, the mother is allowed to interact in a normal way with the child.

N. Merin et al. [27] checked how the children studied in relation with the control group showed a lower fixation in the mother's eyes and the payed more attention to the eye regions. Children who showed alterations had older siblings diagnosed with autism.

Nevertheless,G.S. Young et al. [28] employed this technique in children with six months of age with the aim of checking wether the gaze pattern could be an indicator of a possible risk of autism, but it was proved that no significant evidences between the control group and the ASD group existed, despite the fact that the ASD group maintained the gaze for a longer time in the mouth region. But it was concluded that the more fixation in the mother's mouth region during the experiment predicts a higher level of expressive language as they grow older

- Video

  In 2008 W. Jones et al. [29] Studied how children with autism, before dynamic scenes, observed the mouth region to a greater extent, thus diminishing in the eye region, in comparison to the control group. It is because of this reason why the gaze alteration can be a potential biomedical indicator of the ASD manifestation in an early age . Similarly, the author C.F Norbury [30]also stated that the mouth fixation indicates a higher level of communicative competence within the ASD.

- Multifaceted empathy test

  J.C Kirchner et al. [31], in the year en el año 2011, employed the multifaceted empathy test (MET) method, to evaluate the gaze and the areas of interest in adult people with ASD. To do so, the authors applied the the emotion measurements in the faces and in the identity recognition, and they proved how the ASD group tends to stare less at faces, by means of the conditions of the MET, and the established a correlation between the eye and face fixation time when processing the social skills.

Henceforth, after conducting these studies it has been concluded that the eye and mouth attention is important for the language development [32] as well as the communicative competence, being the gaze patterns an important feature in the social phenotype of the people with autism.

4.2. ASD Gaze Patterns

Since 2002 this technology has been used to study how people with ASD explore by looking the faces or social situations, thus understanding how the visual information is processed. To do so, a series of research works were carried out, where authors and researchers applied static or dynamic scenes.

4.2.1. Static Scenes

By means of static scenes, several studies have been made to evaluate the way people with ASD use the information of the face when making social judgements, checking the relation between the gaze in faces and the social organization of the people with ASD, thus studying how these people process the social information. In the year 2002 the author Van der Gees et al. [33] conducted a study concerning the problem this people have at the time of processing the social information. The studies carried out hitherto associated the particular attitude these people have with social stimuli. But this study evidenced that people with autistic spectrum disorder maintain the gaze before those cartoon images including human figures, and the gaze is similar to those children of the same age and intelligence quotient. That is to say, people with autism do not have specific problems in the visual stimuli processing owning social elements, just as not having found any difference when observing neutral elements. Nevertheless, the author associated the abnormal way of looking in the everyday life to other factors such as the social interaction and not to the nature of social stimuli.

In 2006, and continuing with these studies , M.T Mercadante et al. [34] executed an experiment showing 9 social scenes including human figures (two of them with cat masks) and 3 non social images. People with ASD presented a greater endowment of saccadic movements before the social images in comparison to the control group. This control group, in turn, showed a higher number of fixations in the image corresponding to a woman with a cat mask and blindfolded eyes. The author concluded that there actually are differences in relation to people with ASD at the time of exploring human images.

In the year 2007 the authors M.L Spezio et al. [35], investigated this relation by measuring on the one hand the exploration of faces, and, on the other hand, the way the facial areas were really used during social judgements. In the experiment 9 adults with a high level of autism took part. This group failed at the time of making use of the information coming from the eye regions, thus trusting the mouth information.

D.M Riby et al. [36] in 2009, combined exercises (link an element with its name) with the information obtained from the eye tracker, where the ASD group focused the most when executing and completing the exercises. A significant difference was found between the control group and the group with autism, which could lead to differences at the time of executing the activities [37].Although no significant differences were found in the duration of the gaze in the objective items, people with ASD needed more time to complete the different exercise, and focused more in the regions of images to complete the task.

By means of the eyetracker some visual attention aspects were also evaluated [38] together with the repetitive behaviour in people with ASD, evaluated with children with typical development. To do so, static images with non-social content were used, including among these elements of interest or known by the children such as trains, furniture images with social content. In the study they checked how the attention was more limited, more detail oriented and more perseverant in the group of autism. The results indicated the fact that children with with autism have a general pattern of atypical visual attention, thus showing a tendency to persevere in the images of interest and focusing on details. Aligned with this study, the author Shic et al. [39] employed static images of faces to evaluate the entropy of the scanning patterns in order to be able to characterize the attention of children with ASD by means of faces. In this study, children between 2 and 4 years of age took part, with and without ASD, and some differences were found in the gaze patterns of people with ASD and people with a neurotypical development., both in the regions of interest of the faces and in the gaze patterns with respect to the whole face altogether.

There exist a series of studies in which, In addition to the evaluation of the route, gaze fixation, the behaviour of the pupil in the people with ASD was also checked. People with ASD show a contraction in the pupil when observing people's faces whereas the control group tend to show a dilation of the pupil [40] [41].

4.2.2. Dynamic Scenes

One of the preliminary studies conducted with the eye tracking technology and moving images, was carried out by Amy klin et al. [42] in the year 2002.On it, several videos in which complex social scenes and different distractors elements appeared were used. 4 regions of interest were analysed: mouth, eyes, body and objects. Just as in the aforementioned studies, it was proved the way people with autism did not fix the gaze in the character's eyes. In fact, it was stated that they maintain the gaze two times more in the body and area, and in the area of the objects appearing on scene than the control group. It was checked how the main indicator of autism is the less fixation time in the eye region [43]. Additionally, the fixation in the mouth and in the objects is correlated to the social functioning; That is to say, a greater concentration in mouth predicted a better social adaptation, and a less autistic social decay, whereas more time over the objects predicted the opposite relation. Consequently, in social situations, the individuals with autism show abnormal patterns maintaining less time staring at the region of the eyes, and increasing in the mouth, body and objects. It was therefore defined as the gazing time in the mouth and objects, and not in the eyes, as a strong indicator of the degree of social competence.

This very same year, the author C. Trepagnier et al. [44] checked by means of a little experiment showing stereoscopic images and applying the virtual reality technology and the eye tracking technology the way people with Asperger showed a lower fixation in the central part of the face in comparison to the control group, which lead the authors to stablish how these people have a disability at the time of processing and evaluating the information on the faces. M-Freeth et al. [45] used photographies with complex scenes. Either the control group and the ASD group focused over a similar period of time on the face during both scenes. Nonetheless, differences were met among the attention priorities in the region of face containing the eyes. Besides, despite the fact that people with ASD turned the attention to the gaze of the person on scene, the attention in the place where the people on scene fixed the gaze; It did not increase, as it was the case of the group with neutotypical development.

In the year 2009,O. Grynszpan et al. [46] evaluated the capacity of facial information processing during a conversation, taking as a hypothesis the fact that the difficulty to appreciate the synergy between the facial expressions and the speed could be related with the alterations provoked when diverting the attention between them. By means of virtual reality environments and eye tracking, it ws intended to compensate the deficit in the change of attention allocated to autism, and applying it as a part of the therapies.

People with ASD possess difficulties in the skills related with the imitation of actions , specially at the time of imitating gestures with non- meaningful actions in relation to meaningful actions. G. Vivanti et al. [47] evaluated the capacity of imitation in these people by means of visual attention similar to the control group, but the attention diminished in the face of the model to be imitated. Besides, these people showed a lower precision when imitating the two evaluated types (the visual attention in the actions displayed was related with the imitation precision in the non-significant gestures).

Furthermore, the forming of prototypes with natural faces was also studied, thus concluding that the difficulty of image processing is related with the prototype abstraction form [48] and not due to attention factors, inasmuch as there is no difference in the overall face attention patterns [49]

5. Conclusion

The studies conducted in relation to the eye tracking of the people with ASD have been guided by two types of tests: videos with social scenes or static images of individuals, and it has been proven the way greater differences are appreciated between the control group and the people affected by ASD, more particularly in the dynamic stimuli including social scenes. On them, the fixation in the regions of the eye diminishes, thus increasing in the regions of the body. After these studies, an important aspect that has been detected is that the users' fixation on the mouth is a feature presented by people with ASD in the field of social competences. [50]. In addition, people with ASD maintain the gaze over less time in the face region that people with a neurotypical development [51]. Thus being defined as an element predictive of the social response measurement of these people [52].

Despite of the authors that state that no differences are appreciate between the total amount of time in the observation of eyes, mouth, they actually determine that people with autism tend to look over less time the region of the eyes in comparison to those people with neurotypical development [53] [54].Nevertheless, the paradigms used thus far are incorrect due to the fact that they do not present social information in a real environment [55]. Another problem being encountered here is the diversity of the tests carried out by means of static scenes, photographs, association exercises and the mixed results obtained from these experiments. It is due to this reason why, in the following research works, it is intended to undertake a study in which the behaviour of people with autism is determined by using social scenes evaluating the areas of interest (eyes, mouth, objects and body), fixation time and pupil, together with the comprehension of the social situation to be studied.

References

[1] M. B. Carmona, M. P. la Paz, J. Artigas-Pallarés, R. H. Zúñiga, M. I. Aletxa, J. Martos-Pérez, F. Mulas, J. Muñoz-Yunta, S. Palacios, J. Tamarit, and J. Valdizán, "Guía de buena práctica para la investigación de los trastornos del espectro autista," *Revista de neurología. IF 2011:0.790 (Q4 165/192)*, vol. 41, no. 6, pp. 371–377, 2005.

[2] E. Álvarez Alcantara, "Trastornos del espectro autista," *Revista Mexicana de Pediatria*, vol. 74, no. 6, pp. 269 – 276, 2007.

[3] T. Thompson, "Autism research and services for young children: History, progress and challenges," *Journal of Applied Research in Intellectual Disabilities*, vol. 26, no. 2, pp. 81–107, 2013.

[4] S. L. Gómez, R. M. R. Torres, and E. M. T. Ares, "Revisiones sobre el autismo," *Revista Latinoamericana de Psicología*, vol. 41, no. 3, pp. 555–570, 2009.

[5] L. F. Repeto, Ed., *El síndrome de Asperger en adultos*, 2010.

[6] F. B. Rivera, "Breve revisi'on histórica del autismo," *Revista Asociacón Esp. Neurop-siquiatría*, vol. 27, no. 100, pp. 333–353, 2007.

[7] C. T. Gutiérrez, M. Rodríguez, D. D. L. Rosa, G. Morales, and A. V. V. Meerbeke, "Caracterizaci'on de niños y adolescentes con trastornos del espectro autista en una institución de bogotá," *Revista Asociacón Esp. Neuropsiquiatría*, vol. 27, no. 02, pp. 90–96, 2011.

[8] L. Wing, "Asperger's syndrome: a clinical account," *Psychological Medicine. IF 2011: 6.159 (Q1 6/75)*, vol. 11, no. 01, pp. 115–129, 1981.

[9] M. de la Iglesia Gutierrez and J. S. O. Parra, Eds., *Autismo y síndrome de As-perger.Trastornos del espectro autista de alto funcionamiento. Guía para educadores y familiares.*   Editorial CEPE, 2007.

[10] G. Lanzy, U. Balottin, C. Zambrino, A. Gerardo, E. Bettaglio, and P. Manfredi, "Com-paración de las sistemas diagnósticos clasificatorios del desarrollo:un estudio de veinte caso," *V Congreso internacional de autismo-europa*, 1998.

[11] L. Wing and J. Gould, "Prevalence of autistic spectrum disorder in the uk: E. from-bonne autism," *SAGE Publications*, vol. 2, no. 1, pp. 227–229, 1997.

[12] J. S. O. Parra and M. B. Carmona, "Ineficacia en la comunicación referencial de per-sonas con autismo y otros trastornos relacionados," *Anuario de Psicología*, vol. 75, pp. 119–146, 1997.

[13] I. Rapin, "The autistic spectrum disorders," *New England Journal of Medicine. IF 2011: 53.298 (Q1:1/155)*, vol. 347, no. 5, pp. 302–303, 2002. [Online]. Available: http://www.nejm.org/doi/full/10.1056/NEJMp020062

[14] M. Stanković, A. Lakić, and N. Ilić, "Autism and autistic spectrum disorders in the context of new dsm-v classification, and clinical and epidemiological data," *Srpski arhiv za celokupno lekarstvo*, vol. 140, no. 3-4, pp. 236–243, 2012.

[15] A. P. Association, Ed., *DSM IV-R Diagnostic and Statistical Manual*, 2000.

[16] J. A. Worley and J. L. Matson, "Comparing symptoms of autism spectrum disorders using the current< i> dsm-iv-tr</i> diagnostic criteria and the proposed< i> dsm-v</i> diagnostic criteria," *Research in Autism Spectrum Disorders*, vol. 6, no. 2, pp. 965–970, 2012.

[17] Y. Hassan Montero and V. Herrero Solana, "Eye-tracking en interacción persona-ordenador," *No solo usabilidad*, no. 6, 2007.

[18] L. R. s. M. Samuel Almeida, Ana Veloso, "The eyes and games: A survey of visual attention and eye tracking input in video games," *Proceedings of SBGames*, 2011.

[19] G. T. Buswell, "How people look at pictures: a study of the psychology and perception in art." *American Psychological Association*, 1935.

[20] D. W. Hansen and Q. Ji, "In the eye of the beholder: A survey of models for eyes and gaze," *Pattern Analysis and Machine Intelligence, IEEE Transactions on*, vol. 32, no. 3, pp. 478–500, 2010.

[21] J. J. Cerrolaza, A. Villanueva, and R. Cabeza, "Study of polynomial mapping functions in video-oculography eye trackers," *ACM Transactions on Computer-Human Interaction (TOCHI). IF 2011:0.838 (Q3 81/135)*, vol. 19, no. 2, p. 10, 2012.

[22] M. Viqueira, B. G. Zapirain, and A. M. Zorrilla, "Ocular movement and cardiac rhythm control using eeg techniques," 2013.

[23] A. Goldberg, J.H.; Wichansky, "Eye tracking in usability evaluation: A practitioner's guide," *Proceedings of SBGames*, 2003.

[24] J. Renshaw, "Understanding visual influence in graph design through temporal and spatial eye movement characteristics," *Interacting with computers*, vol. 16, pp. 557–578, 2004.

[25] L. Granka, T. Joachims, and G. Gay, "Eye-tracking analysis of user behavior," *SIGIR*, p. 25?29, 2004.

[26] Poynter, "Eyetrack iii: online news consumer behavior in age of multimedia," *SIGIR*, p. 25?29, 2004.

[27] N. Merin, G. Young, S. Ozonoff, and S. Rogers, "Visual fixation patterns during reciprocal social interaction distinguish a subgroup of 6-month-old infants at-risk for autism from comparison infants," *Journal of Autism and Developmental Disorders*, vol. 37, no. 1, pp. 108–121, 2007.

[28] G. Young, N. Merin, S. Rogers, and S. Ozonoff, "Gaze behavior and affect at 6 months: Predicting clinical outcomes and language development in typically developing infants and infants at risk for autism," *Developmental science*, vol. 12, no. 5, pp. 798–814, 2009.

[29] W. Jones, K. Carr, and A. Klin, "Absence of preferential looking to the eyes of approaching adults predicts level of social disability in 2-year-old toddlers with autism spectrum disorder," *Archives of General Psychiatry. IF 2011: 12.016 (Q1 3/130)*, vol. 65, no. 8, p. 946, 2008.

[30] C. Norbury, J. Brock, L. Cragg, S. Einav, H. Griffiths, and K. Nation, "Eye-movement patterns are associated with communicative competence in autistic spectrum disorders," *Journal of Child Psychology and Psychiatry. IF 2011:4.281 (Q1 8/75)*, vol. 50, no. 7, pp. 834–842, 2009.

[31] J. Kirchner, A. Hatri, H. Heekeren, and I. Dziobek, "Autistic symptomatology, face processing abilities, and eye fixation patterns," *Journal of autism and developmental disorders IF 3.341*, vol. 41, no. 2, pp. 158–167, 2011.

[32] D. J. Lewkowicz and A. M. Hansen-Tift, "Infants deploy selective attention to the mouth of a talking face when learning speech," *Proceedings of the National Academy of Sciences*, vol. 109, no. 5, pp. 1431–1436, 2012.

[33] J. Van der Geest, C. Kemner, G. Camfferman, M. Verbaten, and H. Van Engeland, "Looking at images with human figures: comparison between autistic and normal children," *Journal of autism and developmental disorders*, vol. 32, no. 2, pp. 69–75, 2002.

[34] M. Mercadante, E. Macedo, P. Baptista, C. Paula, and J. Schwartzman, "Saccadic movements using eye-tracking technology in individuals with autism spectrum disorders: pilot study," *Arquivos de neuro-psiquiatria. IF 2011:0.722 (Q4 225/244)*, vol. 64, no. 3A, pp. 559–562, 2006.

[35] M. Spezio, R. Adolphs, R. Hurley, and J. Piven, "Abnormal use of facial information in high-functioning autism," *Journal of autism and developmental disorders*, vol. 37, no. 5, pp. 929–939, 2007.

[36] D. Riby and M. Doherty, "Tracking eye movements proves informative for the study of gaze direction detection in autism," *Research in Autism Spectrum Disorders*, vol. 3, no. 3, pp. 723–733, 2009.

[37] M. R. Swanson, G. C. Serlin, and M. Siller, "Broad autism phenotype in typically developing children predicts performance on an eye-tracking measure of joint attention," *Journal of Autism and Developmental Disorders*, pp. 1–12, 2012.

[38] N. Sasson, L. Turner-Brown, T. Holtzclaw, K. Lam, and J. Bodfish, "Children with autism demonstrate circumscribed attention during passive viewing of complex social and nonsocial picture arrays," *Autism Research*, vol. 1, no. 1, pp. 31–42, 2008.

[39] F. Shic, K. Chawarska, J. Bradshaw, and B. Scassellati, "Autism, eye-tracking, entropy," in *Development and Learning, 2008. ICDL 2008. 7th IEEE International Conference on.* IEEE, 2008, pp. 73–78.

[40] C. Anderson, J. Colombo, and D. Shaddy, "Visual scanning and pupillary responses in young children with autism spectrum disorder," *Journal of Clinical and Experimental Neuropsychology*, vol. 28, no. 7, pp. 1238–1256, 2006.

[41] T. Falck-Ytter, "Face inversion effects in autism: a combined looking time and pupillometric study," *Autism research*, vol. 1, no. 5, pp. 297–306, 2008.

[42] A. Klin, W. Jones, R. Schultz, F. Volkmar, and D. Cohen, "Visual fixation patterns during viewing of naturalistic social situations as predictors of social competence in individuals with autism," *Archives of general psychiatry. IF 2011: 12.016 (Q1 3/130)*, vol. 59, no. 9, p. 809, 2002.

[43] W. Jones and A. Klin, "System and method for quantifying and mapping visual salience," *Autism dev disorder*, vol. 16, 2012.

[44] C. Trepagnier, M. Sebrechts, and R. Peterson, "Atypical face gaze in autism," *Cyberpsychology & Behavior*, vol. 5, no. 3, pp. 213–217, 2002.

[45] M. Freeth, P. Chapman, D. Ropar, and P. Mitchell, "Do gaze cues in complex scenes capture and direct the attention of high functioning adolescents with asd? evidence from eye-tracking," *Journal of autism and developmental disorders IF 3.341*, vol. 40, no. 5, pp. 534–547, 2010.

[46] O. Grynszpan, J. Nadel, J. Constant, F. Le Barillier, N. Carbonell, J. Simonin, J. Martin, and M. Courgeon, "A new virtual environment paradigm for high functioning autism intended to help attentional disengagement in a social context bridging the gap between relevance theory and executive dysfunction," in *Virtual Rehabilitation International Conference, 2009*.   IEEE, 2009, pp. 51–58.

[47] G. Vivanti, A. Nadig, S. Ozonoff, S. Rogers *et al.*, "What do children with autism attend to during imitation tasks?" *Journal of experimental child psychology*, vol. 101, no. 3, p. 186, 2008.

[48] M. Freeth, D. Ropar, P. Mitchell, P. Chapman, and S. Loher, "Brief report: how adolescents with asd process social information in complex scenes. combining evidence from eye movements and verbal descriptions," *Journal of autism and developmental disorders IF 2001 3.341*, vol. 41, no. 3, pp. 364–371, 2011.

[49] H. Gastgeb, D. Wilkinson, N. Minshew, and M. Strauss, "Can individuals with autism abstract prototypes of natural faces?" *Journal of autism and developmental disorders IF 3.341*, vol. 41, no. 12, pp. 1609–1618, 2011.

[50] Z. Boraston and S. Blakemore, "The application of eye-tracking technology in the study of autism," *The Journal of physiology*, vol. 581, no. 3, pp. 893–898, 2007.

[51] D. Riby and P. Hancock, "Looking at movies and cartoons: eye-tracking evidence from williams syndrome and autism," *Journal of Intellectual Disability Research*, vol. 53, no. 2, pp. 169–181, 2009.

[52] L. Speer, A. Cook, W. McMahon, and E. Clark, "Face processing in children with autism effects of stimulus contents and type," *Autism*, vol. 11, no. 3, pp. 265–277, 2007.

[53] C. Anderson and J. Colombo, "Larger tonic pupil size in young children with autism spectrum disorder," *Developmental psychobiology. IF 2011:2.977 (Q2 17/40)*, vol. 51, no. 2, pp. 207–211, 2009.

[54] J. Wagner, S. Hirsch, V. Vogel-Farley, E. Redcay, and C. Nelson, "Eye-tracking, autonomic, and electrophysiological correlates of emotional face processing in adolescents with autism spectrum disorder," *Journal of Autism and Developmental Disorders*, pp. 1–12, 2012.

[55] S. Fletcher-Watson, S. Leekam, V. Benson, M. Frank, and J. Findlay, "Eye-movements reveal attention to social information in autism spectrum disorder," *Neuropsychologia. IF 2011:3.636 (Q1 7/48)*, vol. 47, no. 1, pp. 248–257, 2009.

In: Advances in Medicine and Biology. Volume 69   ISBN: 978-1-62808-088-9
Editor: Leon V. Berhardt   © 2013 Nova Science Publishers, Inc.

Chapter VIII

Evolution and Use of Serious Games for Health: Review and Practical Case about People with ADHD

Maite Frutos-Pascual,[*] *Begoña Garcia Zapirain*[†]
Deusto-Tech Life, University of Deusto, Bilbao, Spain

This chapter explains the thematic of Serious Games, and specially their application in the field of health and their exploitation within the collective of Attention Deficit Hyperactivity Disorder (ADHD) which is one of the most prevalent childhood disorders. The key point in the development of children diagnosed with ADHD is to enhance motivation and engagement towards academic activities and therapies. *Serious Games for Health* could be a complementary solution constituting a powerful tool that fosters engagement and motivation in therapies combining video game technologies with therapies. Even though some studies are focused on the evidence of possible adverse effects related to the misuse or abuse of videogames in children diagnosed with ADHD; there are videogames that boost and enhance key features in the development of these diagnosed children and teenagers. This chapter gives an historical contextualization of this trend and reviews the markets available, as well as studies its application within the field of the Attention Deficit Hyperactivity Disorder (ADHD) and reviews the trend analysis in this field. As a final conclusion it could be stated that the use game based therapies in junction with other technologies for therapy customization in real time could be an effective way of therapy in its use in children and teenagers diagnosed with ADHD .

[*]E-mail address: maitefrutos@deusto.es
[†]E-mail address: mbgarciazapi@deusto.es

Keywords: Serious Games for Health; ADHD; Evolution; Use; Review.

1. Introduction

Attention Deficit Hyperactivity Disorder (ADHD) is one of the most prevalent childhood disorders. It affects around the 5.29% of the worldwide population [1]. These statistics are steadily rising due to the increase of children diagnosed with ADHD. The most significant increment took place in the United States, where children diagnosed with ADHD have been tripled during the last thirty years, reaching the number of 35 per thousand in the late 90s, and still growing today [2].

The ADHD collective presents bigger difficulties in learning than the rest of children population [3]. In general, this academic performance is due to the difficulties this collective has with time management, tasks, prioritizing, keeping sustained attention and controlling their answers and impulses, as well as enhancing their cognitive abilities in the scholarly field.

When this Attention Deficit Disorder Diagnosis is severe, it is usual that it leads to scholar failure. In order to fight against this, it is necessary to obtain an additional effort from every person involved in the development of the diagnosed child. It is important to understand what exactly the disorder is, what it entails and which the consequences are in medium term if there are no appropriate measurements taken.

The key point in the development of children diagnosed with ADHD is enhancing motivation and engagement towards academic activities and therapies. It is necessary to boost their learning and memory skills, concentration, attention and time management using structured activities with specific guidelines and effective materials. One of the available solutions is to motivate interest and engagement of this collective towards these activities. The use of this conjunction with an early intervention can lead to the reduction of conductual problems and their negative consequences in the medium term.

Game-based Learning and Serious Games for Health could be a complementary solution and constitutes a powerful tool that fosters engagement and motivation in therapies. These solutions provide incremental levels of challenge and the opportunity to learn and understand some rules while performing specific actions. They also constitute a convincing environment for learning and therapies [4].

These characteristics constitute a step forward in the enhancement of school performance and the reinforcement of skills in children diagnosed with ADHD. This could be also extended to other collectives. Paraphrasing Seymour's Paper the problem of educational system is not that school abilities are hard or specially demanding but that they are in general boring and difficult to keep children engaged to them [5]. This game-based solution can be encompassed under the Serious Games concept, review that encompasses the objective of this chapter.

Before defining the Serious Games term, it is convenient to adopt a proper definition and contextualization of the plain term Game. Through the years, this terminology has been granted with many definitions. Authors' favourite is the one explained in detail in Jane McGonigal's book Reality is Broken: Why Games Make Us Better and How They Can Change The World [6]. She explains Games as the junction of four main characteristics:

- **Objective:** Every game has a main goal, which is what players should be focused on.

- **Rules:** Limitation or guidelines that players should follow in order to achieve the main goal.

- **Feedback:** At which point is the player from the target. This is generally shown as levels, punctuations, point or progress bars.

- **Voluntary participation:** Every player has to accept conscious and voluntarily the goal, rules and feedback of the game.

The videogame industry is a booming industry valued at 25 billion dollars, where the mean age of the average player is 37 years old and the average time he/she has invested playing is around 12 years [7].

Since the early stages of the 21st century, the videogame industry is established as a consolidated market inside the culture and day-to-day living of users. Videogame accessibility and prosperity is due to the diversity of technologies and the genres available on it. This diversity comprises the breeding ground for new tendencies using this potential. One of these trends is the Serious Games for Health one that is defined in the following paragraphs and contextualized and analyzed along this chapter.

As far as its functional definition is concerned, every Serious Games is based on the four main pillars defined, and it also complies with the premise that its ultimate goal goes beyond entertainment, leaving a further residue of knowledge, skill, routine habit or other capacity in the player.

With respect to its technical definition, it can be stated that Serious Games are the application of state-of-the-art technologies, processes, and designs commonly used in the videogame industry to give a solution to specific issues in the society. It is also important to mention that Serious Games promotes the transfer and reuse of know-how, processes, developments and techniques used in videogames to other environments where traditionally these technologies are not used [8].

This chapter outlines a historical contextualization of the *Serious Games* trend, followed by classification of the available markets, as well as the analysis, study and application of them within the field of the Attention Deficit Hyperactivity Disorder (ADHD).

2. History

The *Serious Games* term was started by North American researcher Clark Abt in his book "Serious Games" in the 70s [9]. Abt worked as a researcher in an American laboratory during the cold war. One of his main objectives was the evaluation of games usage in training and education.

During the beginnings of the digital videogame age, there were other references to the term "Serious Games" in the literature. One of those is the one included in the book *"The New Alexandria Simulation: A Serious Game of State and Local Politics"* in 1973. This book was centered in explaining a game designed for teaching the basis of the politics system in the United States [10].

During the Cold War (1947 - 1991), the U.S. military system invested a lot of economic resources in technological improvements that would come later massively to households, but that initially had a military purpose. One of this technological developments was the use of simulations and war games for military training [11].

One example of these computer-based military games was *HUTSPIEL*, created in 1955 as a strategy game that allows players to experiment the impact of military weapons in a world war. Three years later, in 1958, it was launched *THEATERSPIEL*, as a further developed version of *HUTSPIEL* [12].

In the sixties, a special division was developed for the study and development of games with military purposes, the *"Joint War Games Agency"* [13]. This leads to the birth of lots of games with training and strategy purposes such as *T.E.M.P.E.R*, led by the aforementioned Clark Abt [14], *CARMONETTE* [15], *NEWS*, among others.

Leaving aside the purely military matters, in other areas also began to lay the foundations of the Serious Games trend [16], but with less impact.

In **educational** field, one of the most famous projects was *"The Oregon Trail"*, launched in 1971. It was designed by three American history teachers, and it was developed as a "only text" game [17]. It was a big success for teaching American history in the classroom. Due to this success, there were launched lots of expansions, sequels and spin-offs such as *"The Oregon Trail II"* [18]; *"The Oregon Trail 3rd Edition"*; *"The Amazon Trail"* and *"The Africa Trail"*.

In the **health** field, pioneer *Serious Games* were focused on learning. *Captain Novolin* was developed to teach children to deal with diabetes and for the management and control of their sugar levels through the use of a diabetic superhero [19]. *Packy & Marlon* came up as a multigamer adaptation of the previous outlined game [20].

In the **art** and **culture** field, *Versailles 1685* [21] is the insignia of the cultural entertainment movement. After this, there were lots of titles launched and set in different periods and civilizations: *Egypt 1156 BC Tomb of the pharaoh*; *Byzantine: The Betrayal*; *China, the Forbidden City*; *Pilgrim Faith As a Weapon*; *Vikings*; *Rome: Caesar's Will*; among others [16].

In the **publicity** field, also known as *advergames*, many alimentary brands have being using videogames as a tool for marketing purposes, such as *Kool Aid Man*; *M.C. Kids*; *Chex Quest*; among others.

However, the **official starting point** of current *Serious Games* movement has its origin in the 4th of July of 2002, the Independence Day of the United States. It was in this date when the American army handed out for free the *America's Army* game. This game was based on American army's strategy and simulation missions. It is oriented towards the promotion of the U.S army's reputation among youngsters, and it was also used as a recruitment tool [22]. By 2004 it had been downloaded over 17 million times [23].

During the last decade, *Serious Games* tendency has been consolidated. First, it was established the *Serious Games Initiative* in 2002 and later the *Serious Games Association*.

Since then it was organized numerous meetings, conferences and congresses that entails every market available under the *Serious Games* term. Some of the relevant conferences in this field are the *Game Developers Conference, International Conference on Serious Games and Applications for Health (SeGAH), Serious Games and Social Connect, Serious Play Conference* or *Fun and Serious Games Festival*, among others. Moreover they have

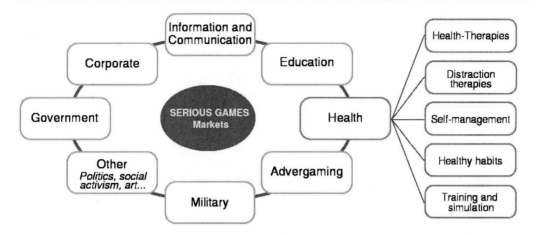

Figure 1. *Serious Games*: Available markets

combined the most advanced techniques in development of *Serious Games* along with other technological advances such as biofeedback or virtual reality, emerging several projects that combine them.

Currently, the flow of Serious Games is a consolidated solution that achieves specific objectives, boosting the immersion and encouraging user involvement into exercises, simulation and therapies. Despite this, the concept of Serious Games can be disproved, so it is vital to maintain the balance between entertainment and final aim, being the first in danger many times. One of the tendencies nowadays is to establish the design methodology necessary to meet these objectives [24] and the use of additional objective measurements such as biofeedback to boos immersion and adaptability in games and to adapt them to final users' necessities [25].

3. Classification of Serious Games

Serious Games industry can be divided into eight different segments or markets, each of them oriented towards a target audience and with a specific and different objective. Figure 1 shows these different areas. Following paragraphs give a brief description of each of them.

- **Health** field, topic of great interest in this chapter, can be divided into several thematics and applications inside *Serious Games*. Some of these different topics are outlined below [26].

  1. **Distraction therapies:** Much research had been made to prove that pain intensity is related with the attention that is paid to it. Several studies have been conducted about the efficacy of videogames and virtual reality in these patients, in order to mitigate pain through the distraction of symptoms.

  2. **Self-management:** These games constitute a key element in the treatment of chronic diseases such as asthma or diabetes. There are games oriented towards

teaching patients to adjust their daily routines and habits to the circumstances of their disorder. Examples of these are *Watch, Discover, Think, and Act* for asthma [27], [28], or for diabetes management *Packie & Marlon* [20] and *Glucoboy* [29], among others.

3. **Healthy habits:** This range includes the *exergames*, games that foster fitness, exercise and games oriented towards teaching healthy habits concerning diets and daily routines. *Squire's Quest*, for the promotion of knowledge about nutritional values [30]; *Dance, Dance Revolution (DDR)*, launched in Japan in 1991; or the commercial releases *Wii Fit* (2007) or *Kinect Sports* (2010) constitute some of the examples in this field.

4. **Training and Simulation:** The junction between virtual reality and medicine can be found in training and simulation environments available for the training of medical staff. Examples of this category are *Pulse!! Virtual Clinical Learning Lab for Health Care Training* [31]. However, despite the abundance of these environments, the necessary characteristics to be considered a Serious Game are not always met.

5. **Health - Therapies:** This series focuses on games as therapy. Inside this research line it can be found several trends oriented towards the diagnosis, phobia treatment, self-discovery and enhancement of specific abilities. In this field they are used turnkey systems as well as commercial adaptations. Some examples of the latter category are *Second Life*, *The Journey to Wild Divine* or *Midtown Madness*.

— **Education:** Educational games are not a newbie trend; it has been used since the ancient Greece. From the 2000 onwards, the market related to education experienced a boom, not only it has been accepted in scholar system but also the availability of toys, games and educational software have increased, leading to the adoption of the *edutainment* term in both scholar and house environments.

— **Advergaming:** Marketing games that allow brands to promote products and services through the use of games. They are commonly used as a complement to other tools such as *e-commerce*.

— **Corporate:** Corporations are developing and increasing interest towards the use of *Serious Games* at workplaces. These games are used to enhance specific skills or as a mean to *gamification* for the promotion of engagement and dedication of employees to the corporation.

— **Information and communication:** They transfer information and messages of different kinds. *Technocity*, for the promotion of technical university degrees; *Interactive Nights Out*, for the prevention of drug consumption, unwanted pregnancy and Sexually Transmitted Diseases (STDs) among teenagers between 17-25 years old; *Food Force*, developed in order to highlight humanitarian problems; *Darfur is dying*, a criticism to geopolitical conflicts; among others.

- **Government:** This market is mainly focused on spreading practical information for citizens, public management politics, and promotion of ethic and civic behaviours. This market also comprises the games based on simulations for training public services works such as *Port of Rotterdam Incident Configurator, Fire Brigade Commander Training, Company Safety Officer Training, 3D Wild Land Fire Simulation* [26].

- **Military:** This market is one of the pioneers inside the Serious Games trend and it is also one of the most extended and used inside it.

- **Others:** Areas such as politics, social activism, religion and art also increased their interest in *Serious Games*. Some examples are outlined thereupon. In politics: *Howard Dean for Iowa, Take Back Illinois*, or moving towards social activism, *September 12th* [32], *PeaceMaker*, which is a simulation of the Israel-Palestinian conflict [33], *A Force More Powerful* for teaching non-violent strategies for the political change [34], *Escape for Woomera's*, that recreates the conditions and environment of the reception and processing centre for immigrants in Woomera [35].

4. The use of Serious Games for Health in ADHD

Reviewing literature, there are several authors who have focused their research on the assessment of potential effects, positive and negative, of the use of videogames both commercial and therapeutic in ADHD. This section presents and analyses the most relevant ones At this point, it is important to distinguish within the analysed studies between commercial videogames and *Serious Games for Health* specially designed for the evaluation, diagnosis or a tool for therapies in children diagnosed with ADHD. This latter category has aroused the attention of scholar centres and therapists during the last years. The reason for this interest is the fact that many children who do not inhibit their hyperactive, impulsive and/or inattentive behaviour in other contexts, are able to regulate this behaviors while playing video games that motivate and engage them, thus encouraging their concentration [36] [37]. Related to commercial videogames, it seems to be some evidence on the vulnerability of certain subgroups within the ADHD diagnosis to videogaming addiction [38] [39]. However, recent studies also suggest that there is no direct relation between exposure to videogames and attention problems, but that there are other risk factors such as inadequate familiar environment or anxiety problems [40]. There are also other researchers that have found some relation between attention and time management skills problems and prolonged videogame exposure [41]. In 2002 Lawrence *et al* conducted a study, which showed that children diagnosed with ADHD resulted on a lower task performance than children in the control group when the exercises or play tasks required a concentration or a higher cognitive process. However, these children perform normally when these games did not require larger working memory or did not involve distractions [42]. Two studies conducted in 2001 (Ferrace-Di, Douglas, Houghton *et al*) and in 2004 (Houghton, Milner *et al*) supported Lawrence's theory about the differences in performance of children diagnosed with ADHD and a control group in commercial games, when they required of an specific working memory load [43] [44].

4.1. Software

This section exposes the implemented solutions in the *Serious Games* field oriented towards children diagnosed with Attention Deficit Hyperactivity Disorder.

4.1.1. Diagnosis and evaluation

The Supermarket Game is a game developed and tested in Brazil. It was designed as an assistant tool for helping in the diagnosis of ADHD. It has proved to be an efficient way to distinguish between children with and without ADHD diagnosis, but it was necessary to keep optimizing its decision-making algorithms to discriminate between different types of ADHD [45] [46]. In 2004, Albert A. Rizzo, Todd Bewerli *et al* have already designed a 3D virtual classroom for helping in the diagnosis of ADHD according to the interaction with the system [47]. *Cyber Cruiser* is a rally-style game oriented towards the evaluation of executive functioning and prospective memory in children with ADHD. It has been used to determine different between these skills between diagnosed children and control groups [48] [49]. The enhancement of executive memory has been object of several developments based on games in the recent years, the most actual one is the design and implementation of two *Serious Games* sets: *Cognitive Carnival* and *Caribbean Quest* in 2012, oriented towards enhancing these skills [50] [51].

4.1.2. Treatment

At present, there are evidences through the literature claiming that videogames can contribute to the enhancement, regulation and/or normalization of some of the key symptoms related to ADHD. The first therapeutic videogame that was made available for this purpose was developed by Pope and Bogart in 1996. It consisted on a modification of previously released software by the NASA. This NASA software was launched for training pilots through the use of progressively adaptive interfaces in a computer environment to players' attention levels [52]. In 2001, Pope and Palsson went one step further and conducted a more extensive development of this NASA patent as an intervention for ADHD. They modified commercial games in combination with the use of the measurements obtained from an EEG [53]. *Play Attention* is another neurofeedback based game for enhancement of selective attention, short-coming memory and discriminative cognitive tasks, among others. It is a game that is controlled through users' attention levels [54] These studies support the theory that the use of neurofeedback in junction with game based therapies could be an effective tool for the treatment of ADHD [55]. Other alternatives for the use of biofeedback is *The journey to wild divine*, a 3D virtual world designed to be controlled through the use of biofeedback. It is a game controlled by relaxation techniques, these techniques are very useful for regulation and monitoring of hyperactivity and impulsivity in children and teenagers diagnosed with ADHD [56]. At the end of 2012, in London, a study evaluating self-management skills in children with ADHD started by controlling a virtual helicopter through the measurement of their activity in specific brain areas using Magnetic Resonance Imaging (MRI) [57]. *Self City* was launched in 2008. It is a game oriented towards the enhancement of social skills among teenagers with ADHD and/or Pervasive Developmental Disorder as a 3D virtual world in which the teenager is forced to face diverse situations [58]. Inside not specifically designed games for ADHD but instead oriented towards a wide spectrum of developmental disorders in children and teenagers, there are some examples such as *Play Mancer* and *Personal Investigator (PI)*. *Play Mancer* is a project designed as a European partnership in 2007. It was focused on the creation and design of a new common framework for *Serious Games* for therapies development [59] [60]. *Personal Investigator (PI)* is a 3D environment for helping teenagers with developmental disorder through the use of Focused Solution Therapies (SFT) and games in therapy. Teen players should manage themselves in a virtual environment that is set in a detective academy where they have to solve some quizzes and challenges [61]. Moreover, these games are specifically designed for the diagnosis and/or treatment of ADHD or other disorders. In recent years it has been used adaptations of commercial videogames for ADHD therapy. Inside this category there is the case of *Robomemo (Cogmed)* [62].

5.   Trend analysis

This section analyses current trends related to the analysis, implementation, research and development of serious games, specially oriented towards the health field. From a design standpoint; actual trends in serious games are focused on the research, layout and implantation of design specific methodologies for the development of serious games. These methodologies should link pattern guidelines in order to balance contests with entertainment in such a way that games are not mere simulations and they provide users with fun and engagement tools. This is a global trend in which the main goal is entertainment. The junction of characteristic game elements in videogames with pedagogical elements are the key point for maintaining entertainment and learning in perfect balance. In this area, a research process for principles underlying motivation and design guidelines and structured strategies that should be integrated and used in the design of serious games for health would be needed. [63]. From the point of view of assessing the impact of serious games, the current trend is focused on the need of longitudinal assessment of the impact of serious gaming approaches. This is to examine the effectiveness and real long-term efficiency of these approaches [64]. From a technological perspective, trends in the use of therapeutic video games are geared towards using games with great social interaction, accessible and enjoyable for all ages, and virtual worlds, providing a unique opportunity to wave the narrative content with remote immersive therapies and social interaction between patients and professionals [36]. Games based on social interaction constitute a key point in design and development trends for serious games. The possibility to create online communities enables the transfer of knowledge and experiences between users with similar characteristics. Moreover, and applying this area to the Serious Games for Health field, this social games could boost the creation of new patient-doctor links, transporting therapies, consultations and diagnosis to household environments and making them much more dynamic. Engagement in therapies is greater through the use of these technologies, and users could work collaboratively for a common goal. The junction of these social environments with virtual worlds is a step forward in the immersion of therapies and in the involvement of patients and doctors into therapies. These genres can be used for training and testing therapies, and provide a platform for unlimited social interaction. This trend of *Serious Games* for health also provide the scientific and medical community with a powerful assisted tool for helping in diagnosis, treatment and research of disorders. These communities could take advantage of the collaborative effort.

6.   Conclusion

Attention Deficit Hyperactivity Disorder is one of the disorders with higher prevalence among children and teenagers. It could also affect to academic performance and to the familiar environment of children with this diagnosis. In recent years there have been numerous therapies, which, along with traditional therapies, offer new possibilities for the improvement of characteristic symptoms related to ADHD as attention, executive memory or time management skills. Getting to motivate the interest of ADHD diagnosed children, towards academic activities there is a key point in their development. It is necessary to boost their learning and memory skills, concentration, attention and time management abilities through the use of structured activities, with clear guidelines and using flashy materials. One of the possible solutions for these improvements, as it has been outlined during this chapter, is to arouse the interest of this group through the use of specific games designed for them. As it has been explained in this chapter, some studies are focused on the evidence of possible adverse effects related to the misuse or abuse of videogames in children diagnosed with Attention Deficit Disorder. These effects are specially related to addictive behaviors or excessive sensorial load. However, there are videogames that boost and enhance skills specially related to strategy development, pattern recognition, structured guidelines, and that foster concentration, and time management skills and abilities. All of these characteristics are key features in the development of children and teenagers with ADHD diagnosis. *Serious Games'* boom conciliate these two aspects, joining the potential available under the videogames and investing it completely in the enhancement of specific abilities, aptitudes and skills in children and teenagers with ADHD diagnosis. Combining the potential of *Serious Games* with new approaches such as biofeedback could provide a step forward to the customization of therapies using games specially adapted to each user's needs. Game goals, guidelines and feedback can be adapted then to users' needs in real time, getting a more accessible and engaged experience. These biofeedback techniques enhance therapy adaptability and represent a key point in the immersion of users to therapies. These measurements taken through the use of specific sensors and biofeedback techniques lead to the adaptation in real time of therapies, and could be oriented towards the junction of users and therapies, so that professionals, family and teachers are convinced that the child is doing the exercises appropriate to their developmental level at the time.

With the booming of this development lines and the junction of *Serious Games for Health*, neurofeedback and ADHD, research and development necessary lines are multiplied. As a final conclusion it could be stated that the use of neurofeedback in combination with game based therapies could be an effective way of therapy in its use in children and teenagers diagnosed with Attention Deficit Hyperactivity Disorder.

References

[1] G. Polanczyk, M. de Lima, B. Horta, J. Biederman, and L. Rohde, "The worldwide prevalence of adhd: a systematic review and metaregression analysis," *American Journal of Psychiatry*, vol. 164, no. 6, pp. 942–948, 2007.

[2] M. Olfson, M. Gameroff, S. Marcus, and P. Jensen, "National trends in the treatment of attention deficit hyperactivity disorder," *American Journal of Psychiatry*, vol. 160, no. 6, pp. 1071–1077, 2003.

[3] T. Spencer *et al.*, "Adhd and comorbidity in childhood." *The Journal of clinical psychiatry*, vol. 67, p. 27, 2006.

[4] R. Sandford and B. Williamson, "Games and learning," *NESTA Futurelab*, 2005.

[5] M. Prensky and M. Prensky, "Digital game-based learning," 2008.

[6] J. McGonigal, *Reality is broken: Why games make us better and how they can change the world.* Penguin Press HC, 2011.

[7] E. S. Association *et al.*, "Essential facts about the computer and video game industry. retrieved july 26, 2011," 2011.

[8] T. Susi, M. Johannesson, and P. Backlund, "Serious games: An overview," 2007.

[9] C. Abt Klark, "Serious games," 1970.

[10] D. R. Jansiewicz, *The New Alexandria simulation: a serious game of state and local politics.* Canfield Press, 1973.

[11] E. Halter, *From Sun Tzu to xbox: War and video games.* Thunder's Mouth Press, 2006.

[12] J. O. Harrison Jr and M. F. Barrett, "Computer-aided information systems for gaming," DTIC Document, Tech. Rep., 1964.

[13] A. Banister, "The case for cold war gaming in the military services," *Air University Review*, 1967.

[14] C. C. Abt and M. Gorden, "Report on project temper," *Theory and Research on the Causes of War. Englewood Cliffs: Prentice-Hall, Inc*, 1969.

[15] L. Dondero, "A hierarchy of combat analysis models," *General Research Corporation, USA*, 1973.

[16] D. Djaouti, J. Alvarez, J.-P. Jessel, and O. Rampnoux, "Origins of serious games," *Serious Games and Edutainment Applications*, pp. 25–43, 2011.

[17] D. Rawitsch, B. Heinemann, and P. Dillenberger, "The oregon trail," *HP TSB*, 1971.

[18] M. E. C. Consortium *et al.*, "The oregon trail ii," 1994.

[19] P. Frieberger, "Video game takes on diabetes superhero captain novolin offers treatment tips," *San Francisco Examiner,(Jun. 26, 1992), Fourth Edition, Business Section B*, vol. 1.

[20] S. Brown, D. A. Lieberman, B. Gemeny, Y. Fan, D. Wilson, and D. Pasta, "Educational video game for juvenile diabetes: results of a controlled trial," *Informatics for Health and Social Care*, vol. 22, no. 1, pp. 77–89, 1997.

[21] C. Interactive, "Versailles 1685," *Jogo eletrônico. França*, 1997.

[22] D. Nieborg, "America's army: More than a game," 2004.

[23] J. Alvarez and L. Michaud, "Serious games. advergaming, edugaming, training and more," *IDATE, Monpellier*, 2008.

[24] I. Marfisi-Schottman, S. George, and F. Tarpin-Bernard, "Tools and methods for efficiently designing serious games," in *Proceedings of the 4th Europeen Conference on Games Based Learning ECGBL*, 2010, pp. 226–234.

[25] P. M. Kato, "Video games in health care: Closing the gap." *Review of General Psychology*, vol. 14, no. 2, p. 113, 2010.

[26] D. R. Michael and S. Chen, *Serious games: games that educate, train and inform.* Course Technology PTR, 2006.

[27] L. Bartholomew, R. Gold, G. Parcel, D. Czyzewski, M. Sockrider, M. Fernandez, R. Shegog, and P. Swank, "Watch, discover, think, and act: evaluation of computer-assisted instruction to improve asthma self-management in inner-city children," *Patient Education and Counseling*, vol. 39, no. 2, pp. 269–280, 2000.

[28] L. Bartholomew, R. Shegog, G. Parcel, R. Gold, M. Fernandez, D. Czyzewski, M. Sockrider, and N. Berlin, "Watch, discover, think, and act: a model for patient education program development," *Patient Education and Counseling*, vol. 39, no. 2, pp. 253–268, 2000.

[29] S. G. Slater, "New technology device: Glucoboy®, for disease management of diabetic children and adolescents," *Home Health Care Management & Practice*, vol. 17, no. 3, pp. 246–247, 2005.

[30] T. Baranowski, J. Baranowski, K. W. Cullen, T. Marsh, N. Islam, I. Zakeri, L. Honess-Morreale, and C. demoor, "Squire's quest!: dietary outcome evaluation of a multimedia game," *American journal of preventive medicine*, vol. 24, no. 1, pp. 52–61, 2003.

[31] C. L. Johnston and D. Whatley, "Pulse!!-a virtual learning space project," *Studies in Health Technology and Informatics*, vol. 119, p. 240, 2005.

[32] P. R. Games, "September 12th," 2003.

[33] A. Burak, E. Keylor, and T. Sweeney, "Peacemaker: A video game to teach peace," *Intelligent technologies for interactive entertainment*, pp. 307–310, 2005.

[34] J. Schollmeyer, "shots from a force more powerful," 2006.

[35] K. Wild *et al.*, "Escape from woomera."

[36] N. Wilkinson, R. Ang, and D. Goh, "Online video game therapy for mental health concerns: A review," *International Journal of Social Psychiatry*, vol. 54, no. 4, pp. 370–382, 2008.

[37] H. Geurts, M. Luman, and C. Van Meel, "What's in a game: the effect of social motivation on interference control in boys with adhd and autism spectrum disorders," *Journal of Child Psychology and Psychiatry*, vol. 49, no. 8, pp. 848–857, 2008.

[38] S. Bioulac, L. Arfi, and M. Bouvard, "Attention deficit/hyperactivity disorder and video games: A comparative study of hyperactive and control children." *European Psychiatry*, 2008.

[39] J. Frölich, G. Lehmkuhl, M. Döpfner *et al.*, "[computer games in childhood and adolescence: relations to addictive behavior, adhd, and aggression]," *Zeitschrift Fur Kinder-Und Jugendpsychiatrie Und Psychotherapie*, vol. 37, no. 5, p. 393, 2009.

[40] C. Ferguson, "The influence of television and video game use on attention and school problems: A multivariate analysis with other risk factors controlled," *Journal of psychiatric research*, vol. 45, no. 6, pp. 808–813, 2011.

[41] A. Tolchinsky and S. Jefferson, "Problematic video game play in a college sample and its relationship to time management skills and attention-deficit/hyperactivity disorder symptomology," *Cyberpsychology, Behavior, and Social Networking*, vol. 14, no. 9, pp. 489–496, 2011.

[42] V. Lawrence, S. Houghton, R. Tannock, G. Douglas, K. Durkin, and K. Whiting, "Adhd outside the laboratory: Boys' executive function performance on tasks in videogame play and on a visit to the zoo," *Journal of Abnormal Child Psychology*, vol. 30, no. 5, pp. 447–462, 2002.

[43] S. Houghton, N. Milner, J. West, G. Douglas, V. Lawrence, K. Whiting, R. Tannock, and K. Durkin, "Motor control and sequencing of boys with attention-deficit/hyperactivity disorder (adhd) during computer game play," *British Journal of Educational Technology*, vol. 35, no. 1, pp. 21–34, 2004.

[44] A. Farrace-Di Zinno, G. Douglas, S. Houghton, V. Lawrence, J. West, and K. Whiting, "Body movements of boys with attention deficit hyperactivity disorder (adhd) during computer video game play," *British journal of educational technology*, vol. 32, no. 5, pp. 607–618, 2001.

[45] F. Santos, A. Bastos, L. Andrade, K. Revoredo, and P. Mattos, "Assessment of adhd through a computer game: An experiment with a sample of students," in *Games and Virtual Worlds for Serious Applications (VS-GAMES), 2011 Third International Conference on.* IEEE, 2011, pp. 104–111.

[46] L. Vasconcelos de Andrade, L. Vidal Carvalho, C. Lima, A. Cruz, P. Mattos, C. Franco, A. Soares, and B. Grieco, "Supermarket game: an adaptive intelligent computer game for attention deficit/hyperactivity disorder diagnosis," in *Artificial Intelligence, 2006. MICAI'06. Fifth Mexican International Conference on.* IEEE, 2006, pp. 359–368.

[47] A. A. Rizzo, T. Bowerly, C. Shahabi, J. G. Buckwalter, D. Klimchuk, and R. Mitura, "Diagnosing attention disorders in a virtual classroom," *Computer*, vol. 37, no. 6, pp. 87–89, 2004.

[48] K. A. Kerns, "The cybercruiser: An investigation of development of prospective memory in children," *Journal of the International Neuropsychological Society*, vol. 6, no. 01, pp. 62–70, 2000.

[49] K. A. Kerns and K. J. Price, "An investigation of prospective memory in children with adhd," *Child Neuropsychology*, vol. 7, no. 3, pp. 162–171, 2001.

[50] D. W. Bartle, "Development of cognitive video games for children with attention and memory impairment," Ph.D. dissertation, 2012.

[51] J. Pei and K. Kerns, "Using games to improve functioning in children with fetal alcohol spectrum disorders," *GAMES FOR HEALTH: Research, Development, and Clinical Applications*, 2012.

[52] A. T. Pope and E. H. Bogart, "Method of encouraging attention by correlating video game difficulty with attention level," 1994, uS Patent 5,377,100.

[53] O. S. Palsson, R. L. Harris Sr, and A. T. Pope, "Method and apparatus for encouraging physiological self-regulation through modulation of an operator's control input to a video game or training simulator," 2002, uS Patent 6,450,820.

[54] J. A. Siglin and U. Logic, "Play attention-focusing on success," *Intervention in School and Clinic*, vol. 36, no. 2, pp. 122–124, 2000.

[55] N. Yan, J. Wang, M. Liu, L. Zong, Y. Jiao, J. Yue, Y. Lv, Q. Yang, H. Lan, and Z. Liu, "Designing a brain-computer interface device for neurofeedback using virtual environments," *Journal of Medical and Biological Engineering*, vol. 28, pp. 167–172, 2008.

[56] C. Bell, "The journey to wild divine," 2003.

[57] F. Statements, T. Lives, P. Bear, D. McCall, F. Bruce, D. Harper, K. McCabe, D. Murnaghan, T. Hadley, M. Fry *et al.*, "Helping children affected by disability and infections."

[58] D. van Dijk, R. Hunneman, and S. Wildlevuur, "Self city: Training social skills in a game," in *2nd European Conference on Games Based Learning.* Academic Conferences Limited, 2008, pp. 481–488.

[59] A. Conconi, T. Ganchev, O. Kocsis, G. Papadopoulos, F. Fernández-Aranda, and S. Jiménez-Murcia, "Playmancer: A serious gaming 3d environment," in *Automated solutions for Cross Media Content and Multi-channel Distribution, 2008. AXMEDIS'08. International Conference on.* IEEE, 2008, pp. 111–117.

[60] S. Jiménez-Murcia, F. Fernández-Aranda, E. Kalapanidas, D. Konstantas, T. Ganchev, O. Kocsis, T. Lam, J. J. Santamaría, T. Raguin, C. Breiteneder *et al.*, "Playmancer project: A serious videogame as an additional therapy tool for eating and impulse control disorders," *Annual Review of Cybertherapy and Telemedicine 2009: Advanced Technologies in the Behavioral, Social and Neurosciences*, vol. 144, p. 163, 2009.

[61] D. Coyle, M. Matthews, J. Sharry, A. Nisbet, and G. Doherty, "Personal investigator: A therapeutic 3d game for adolecscent psychotherapy," *Interactive technology and smart education*, vol. 2, no. 2, pp. 73–88, 2005.

[62] T. Klingberg, E. Fernell, P. J. Olesen, M. Johnson, P. Gustafsson, K. Dahlström, C. G. Gillberg, H. Forssberg, and H. Westerberg, "Computerized training of working memory in children with adhd-a randomized, controlled trial," *Journal of the American Academy of Child and Adolescent Psychiatry*, vol. 44, no. 2, pp. 177–186, 2005.

[63] D. Charsky, "From edutainment to serious games: A change in the use of game characteristics," *Games and Culture*, vol. 5, no. 2, pp. 177–198, 2010.

[64] M. F. Young, S. Slota, A. B. Cutter, G. Jalette, G. Mullin, B. Lai, Z. Simeoni, M. Tran, and M. Yukhymenko, "Our princess is in another castle a review of trends in serious gaming for education," *Review of Educational Research*, vol. 82, no. 1, pp. 61–89, 2012.

Index

D

distribution, 2, 14, 15, 50, 76, 82
diversity, vii, 19, 70, 73, 75, 76, 77, 101, 109
DNA, ix, 53, 56, 58, 59, 60, 66
DNA polymerase, 59
DNA sequencing, ix, 53, 66
doctors, 115
dopamine, 8
dorsal horn, 7
dosage, 26, 29
double-blind trial, 32
draft, 93
drug consumption, 112
drug reactions, 25
drugs, 8, 11, 16, 17, 28, 47
DSM, 93, 102
ductus arteriosus, 24, 31

E

ecology, 78, 79, 82
economic damage, ix, 83
ecosystem, 77
ECs, 36, 37, 39, 40, 41, 42, 43
edema, 29
education, 109, 112, 118, 121
educational software, 112
EEG, 114
Egypt, 110
electric field, 10
electrodes, 95
electron, 74
elucidation, 44
embolism, 34
embryogenesis, 14
emission, 94
emotion, 98
emotional distress, 27
empathy, 98
ENA-78, 38
encoding, 57, 58, 61, 62, 85, 87
endangered, viii, 19, 27
endocrine, 2
endothelial cells, 21, 22, 44, 46, 48, 50, 52
endothelial dysfunction, 22, 36
endothelium, 36, 37, 41, 42, 43, 50, 51
endotoxins, 8
energy, 58, 62
engineering, 54, 86
entropy, 99
environments, ix, 13, 70, 73, 76, 77, 79, 80, 81, 100, 101, 105, 108, 109, 112, 113, 114, 115, 116, 120, 121

enzymes, vii, ix, 1, 5, 15, 16, 18, 19, 20, 21, 31, 59, 62, 63, 83, 84, 85, 86, 88
EOG, 95
eosinophils, 42, 43
epidemic, 71
epidemiologic, 24, 32
epidemiologic studies, 24
epidemiology, 77
epidermis, 57, 62
Ergotism, 34
erythrocyte sedimentation rate, 38, 45
ESR, 38, 40, 45
EST, 54, 57, 58, 60, 87
ester, 11, 15
etanercept, 47
etiology, 28, 29
eukaryotic, 85
Europe, 71
evidence, x, 6, 10, 13, 37, 38, 39, 49, 73, 86, 105, 107, 113, 116
evolution, vii, x, 30, 91, 94
executive function, 114, 119
executive functioning, 114
exercise, 15, 24, 25, 32, 34, 99, 112
exercise performance, 25
exploitation, x, 107
exposure, 9, 27, 28, 113
expressed sequence tag, 54, 55, 57, 66
extracellular matrix, 43
extracts, 20
eye movement, 94, 95, 96, 97, 103, 104, 105
eye pattern, x, 91

F

facial expression, 100
families, 38, 85
fantasy, 92
farmers, 54
fat, 31
fatty acids, vii, 1, 2, 19
fever, 2, 8, 9, 10, 13, 14, 37
fibrinolysis, 22
fibrinolytic, 22
fibroblasts, 23, 41, 42, 45, 50
Finland, 76, 79, 81
fish, 16
fitness, 112
fixation, 97, 98, 99, 100, 101, 103, 104
flexibility, 92
flooding, 86
flora, 76
fluid, 11, 12, 43

Q

R

S

U

V

W

Y

Z